HOW TO BE
A *BOSS*
AT AGEING

BOOKS BY ANNIKI SOMMERVILLE

Motherwhelmed

THE HOTBED COLLECTIVE
More Orgasms Please

HOW TO BE
A *BOSS*
AT AGEING

REAL ADVICE ON HOW
TO NAVIGATE AND
EMBRACE MIDLIFE

ANNIKI SOMMERVILLE

Thread

Published by Bookouture in 2021

An imprint of Storyfire Ltd.
Carmelite House
50 Victoria Embankment
London EC4Y 0DZ

www.bookouture.com

ISBN: 978-1-80019-518-9
eBook ISBN: 978-1-80019-516-5

I wrote this book for all the women who are growing older and feeling disillusioned, wobbly and knackered. I hope it helps.

I also wrote this book for my dad, whom I loved more than anything. I would have loved him to read it, even though it wasn't written with him in mind.

CONTENTS

CHAPTER ONE

Should We Really Be Grateful for Simply Being Alive?

Ageing Is Cool Now, Right? What's Your Problem, Old Lady?

If you look in women's magazines or read celebrity interviews, it's easy to feel like women ageing is no longer a big deal. And when I say 'ageing' here I mean *physical ageing* – the way we look as we get older. Later on, I'll come onto all the other aspects like feeling tired, less relevant, struggling to keep up at work, menopause… all those *lovely* things.

Look at any fashion spread in a Sunday supplement, and at least one of the models has long, grey hair and is often in her sixties, at least. The re-vamped *Good Housekeeping* no longer has tips on how to deal with moths eating your cardigans and instead has Davina McCall laughing into the camera wearing a tiny white bikini and showing off her washboard abs and sun-kissed skin. In another spread you might have Goldie Hawn, who is in her seventies. Look at her! She's embracing her imperfections and living life to the full, and she does Pilates at dawn and then takes care of her grandchildren for hours on end and teaches them mindfulness techniques. Where's the problem, ladies? I recently read a quote from the woman herself and she said something about how ageing was good because it meant you were still on the planet.

Now I love Goldie as much as the next celebrity gossip dork, but there is a nagging quibble that comes up for me. So, my question is… Should we really feel grateful for simply being alive? Isn't that setting the bar quite low in terms of life expectations? Forget that I feel like everyone is overtaking me, or that I'm sweating 24/7 and my neck has grown a twin to keep itself company… I'M ALIVE, HOORAH!

Then we have the thorny issue of privilege (and I have plenty of this compared to many, but I don't have Goldie's level – not the house in Malibu or the Pilates teacher on speed dial). Let's also take a moment to absorb the fact that Goldie looks incredible. She looks about fifty, maybe fifty-five, tops. This look feels unobtainable to a woman in her late forties – i.e. ME – let alone a woman in her seventies.

And why are we pretending that this glossy, impossible-to-aspire-to look has been achieved through a bit of Pilates and the odd bunk-up with Kirk Russell? Why isn't anyone discussing how much work goes into looking like Goldie Hawn? There are personal trainers and macrobiotic chefs and facialists and massage therapists, so it probably isn't that much work; but still, a lot of TIME must go into being seventy and looking that way. And what about the discourse around women and ageing? What about the fact that Carol Vorderman is a brilliant mathematician but the newspapers instead call her out on her 'VERY smooth complexion', which is a snide way of saying she's had work done.

Why is there this giant elephant in the room and women are judged if they do something to their faces but are also judged if they age 'naturally' (whatever that means)? Why is it that we don't acknowledge how hard it is for women to navigate getting older when nobody is entirely honest about the physical challenges of getting older in a society that is obsessed with being young?

There is a famous Radiohead video for the song 'Just'. Thom Yorke lies on the ground for the entire video and people walk past and he continues lying on the ground, not moving. This is how I feel most days when I think about ageing. I'm forty-seven, which means I'm nearing fifty. DO YOU HEAR ME, GOD? I AM NEARING FIFTY! I used to go to raves! I used to sing in a Dutch house music band! I once hung out with famous indie bands in Amsterdam and did drugs. I also told a younger colleague about some of these famous indie bands (which can't be named for legal reasons) and realised I sounded just like my dad when he used to talk about bumping into some old blues singer I'd never heard of back in the 1960s, i.e. sad. I remember Gran saying this to me when I was in my early thirties: 'The thing is, Niki, you look in the mirror and you just don't recognise the face staring back at you because you still feel young inside. Inside, I'm a girl of eighteen!'

Gran was amazing, but as her eyesight deteriorated she started to let her beard get very bushy (I suffer with the same affliction but keep it in check with tweezers). I thought she was talking nonsense. Of course, you didn't feel the same when you were that old. And it was sort of nonsense, but I understand it better now. I don't feel forty-seven but I certainly feel more tired and grumpy than I did at eighteen. At eighteen I was basically an empty-headed worrier who obsessed about whether my perm was too curly. When I was eighteen I thought mainly about boys and whether I could afford to buy a packet of cigarettes or a bag of chips (I'm not joking actually – I had no money and usually the fags won).

Let's compare the thought patterns:

Eighteen-year-old me:
I wonder if I should continue growing my fringe out or whether I should get it cut. Would platform shoes suit me? Can I dance in platform shoes? I really fancy that guy Pat, but he has a girlfriend and I have a boyfriend. I wonder if he likes me, because he bit me on the arm the last time we went out. I'm sure there must be something he was trying to tell me. I wonder if my fringe would be better if I swept it up to one side?

Forty-seven-year-old me:
*What the hell kind of job am I going to get that allows me to actu-
ally see my children more than one hour a day? Why is everyone
else so much better at stuff than I am? What if we can't pay the
mortgage anymore? What will we eat if we have no food left in
the fridge? Am I a decent parent? I feel like I'm a lazy parent that
allows the kids to have too much screen time. Will I ever actually
spend my time doing what I want? Why don't I ever have sex
anymore? Why does my body look like a melted candle? What is
the meaning of life? I wonder if my fringe would be better if I
swept it up to one side?*

I have a lot of baggage now. There are parts of that eighteen-
year-old somewhere, but there is also Trauma, Regret, Heartbreak,
Grief. Some happy stuff too, and there's room for more, of course.
We can't just cast it all off and spring about like newborn lambs
(or maybe we can if we believe Goldie Hawn).

One of the classic lines about getting older is the one about
confidence. The one where everyone says how much more confident
they are now that they're older and they don't give a crap about
what people think. This is great in theory and it is how I feel some
of the time, *but* I don't get the impression every woman over forty
is dancing around the beach like a model in a pantyliner advert.

Seventy-five per cent of the time I feel tired, washed up and old.
I start each day doing a body scan and trying to get to grips with
which particular body part will be giving me jip today (usually my
lower back– utterly fucked by childbirth in my forties). I'm haunted
by the idea that the best years are behind me and that those years
weren't particularly good anyway: about four lost to hedonism,
five to studying something I could never get a job doing (working
in TV), then eighteen climbing a greasy, corporate pole trying to
make it to the top of a market research agency, then another five
years struggling to conceive children and miscarrying. Now I'm

child-rearing, nailing it, creating a new career, and being a ballsy old chick, which takes me to the ripe old age of forty-seven (I'm not sure the maths adds up, but you get my gist).

Where does this tiredness come from? Surely you have no reason to be tired. Stop complaining!

If you are one of those chicks who feels like getting older is tickety boo, well this book ain't for you. I respect you, applaud you and wish you all the best (and please message me with how you feel so tickety all the time).

I'm almost fifty and am the mother of two young children. I had my second daughter at forty-six (you stupid twat, I hear you shout) and can't remember a night of unbroken sleep. I'm not alone in the trend to have kids later in life. Statistically, the birth rate is going up amongst women in their forties. There are lots of complicated reasons why this is happening, but for those of us who left it late, the focus can often be on getting pregnant versus how we will cope ONCE we have children. I'm lucky. I know that. There are many women who won't have children but wanted to have them (and there's a chapter on infertility later, as it's something us older women have to face up to).

It's not just children that age us though. It's also the expectations around ageing these days. In some ways, YES, there are reasons to celebrate – women have more equality with men (though there is still a lot of work to be done) and we have more opportunities and choices, especially if we're in a position of privilege. But there is also a lot of pressure: pressure to achieve; to keep going; to look a certain way; to have status; to have a good job; to change the job if you're not happy; to have a social media presence and some sort of digital know-how; to be able to make a boomerang and put subtitles on your Instagram stories; to be a GOOD parent and to excel at parenting and never have a bummer day when you let your standards slip. Even watching the right box sets feels like a competition, plus it's very time consuming. I'm joking, but I always feel Virginia Woolf would have had her enthusiasm for writing dampened if she'd had hours of *Peaky Blinders* to watch each week.

I undertook my own survey of 370 women aged 30–50. Over 50 per cent felt they were more overwhelmed the older they got, and 72 per cent thought they were mainly responsible for the household admin and organisation (which obviously contributes massively to the sense of overwhelm). 'The success of a happy life is to lower your expectations,' someone once told me. It might have been my mother, but I don't want to say it was her because she'll tell me that she never said that and it marks her out as being a pessimist when really she's just pragmatic.

I quickly learnt with small children that lowering expectations was important. If I expected two hours of sleep, then I'd be happy with three. If I expected the floor to be covered with food, then I'd be content with the small square near the door which was clean. The problem is that on a societal level our expectations are sky high. The culture of productivity is not so bad if you're full of energy and a dashing twenty-year-old with a degree in social media, communication and TikTok. It's trickier if you're trying to latch onto the productivity trend with the onset of menopause, a poor body image, a face that makes you weep, no energy and a degree in media from 1997. (That was when I learnt how to edit film footage. I learnt to do it by literally cutting up bits of tape recordings. I am officially qualified to work in a media studio circa 1997 – hoorah!)

The relentless drive to be productive and brilliant is tough, and gets tougher as we age

Part of the problem with ageing for women nowadays is there is no prescribed route. There is no slowing down or expectation to slow down. If anything, the expectation is to put your foot down on the accelerator. No comfy cardigan and a subscription to *Reader's Friend*. No *Arrow* word puzzles whilst slurping on a Murray Mint. Is that why my gran felt eighteen and I feel so old? I spoke to journalist and author Sali Hughes, and she summed up how dramatically the landscape of ageing has changed:

> For our grans' generation, you cut your hair off at forty, and got a cauliflower hair-do at fifty. Look at yourself as an example – you're three years shy of fifty and have a seventeen-month-old daughter, and you're writing a book!

The fact that I was writing a book cheered me up, because writing is something I enjoy and a reason to feel optimistic. And, yes, it feels liberating to have choices nowadays and higher expectations generally. But the flipside is that choice brings pressure to pursue all those choices and to keep up with the culture of busy-ness and productivity which seems to insist that every person fills their time with meaningful activity.

The pressure becomes more intense when the time frame you have to work in becomes ever smaller.

Our grans probably didn't worry too much about whether they were producing interesting social media content or whether they'd managed to launch a new business or whether their kids were as clever as all the other kids or whether they had a satisfying sex life with their partner. I'm not saying life for them was more relaxing – of course there was a tidal wave of sexism that was hard to deal with and women were trapped in their homes while their partners went off strutting about with shoulder pads on or sat in the pub like the Two Ronnies – but it sometimes feels that the continuation of youth and the lack of a clear pathway in terms of what happens when we age, means we just keep trying to keep up with younger people. We keep striving and trying and we are coming up short because we're comparing ourselves to people half our age. Or we're looking at people who are our age and seem to be making no concessions at all to ageing so look the same and act the same and have the kind of punishing regime that would make a twenty-year-old fall over from tiredness.

It's really fucking annoying to read this shit

Here's a sample of the kind of tosh I'm talking about – those articles where they profile someone who is very successful in their forties, and show what they get up to each day:

> **5am:** Get up and do forty-five minutes of HIIT training with my personal trainer.
>
> **5.45am:** Read work emails and then do a conference call with our New York office. Get a B vitamin shot in my arm.
>
> **7.00am:** Get dressed in my cashmere running kit, drink a smoothie and have a breakfast Zoom with my team.
>
> **7:30am:** Work on my laptop whilst running at the same time and developing my health and wellbeing app.
>
> **10:00am:** Teach my children meditation and Latin.
>
> **12:00am:** Eat a plate of almonds and drink water.
>
> **1:00pm:** COLLAPSE INTO A POOL OF TEARS AND TIREDNESS AND HAVE TO PHONE AN AMBULANCE TO TAKE ME AWAY AS I CAN'T STAND THIS SHIT ANYMORE.

We've all read this kind of guff (okay, maybe not the last bit) and we've all thought about why our own lives don't measure up to this kind of punishing regime. As we reach our forties and then go into our late forties, the notion that this kind of lifestyle is desirable, or even feasible, is ridiculous.

Us old birds must cut ourselves some collective slack. We must acknowledge that it's okay to age, that we don't have to punish ourselves or deny that it's happening; that we can't do everything and achieve everything, but can perhaps crystallise what matters most to us (so, it's out with people pleasing and doing what other people say we should do and in with doing what we want and caring less about what other people think).

We should also feel within our rights to reject the culture of busy, busy, busy, because it doesn't serve us. It doesn't actually serve anyone apart from a capitalist society that wants us to consume and produce all the time. Covid-19 has taught us that having lots of followers, or a child that can speak Mandarin whilst doing laps around an Olympic-sized swimming pool, doesn't really matter in the grand scheme of things. There is life and death to consider. We spend much of our time avoiding the death chat, but when we see it happening around us and it becomes a possibility, then our perspectives get shaken up. We have all started thinking about what really matters. Perhaps our lives flashed before our eyes a little. That busy, busy culture looks a bit foolish in light of Covid-19. Like everyone is a participant in one of those 24-hour charity dancing marathons and is about to collapse in a heap.

So, there is a lesson about slowing down and being more mindful, about recalibrating and considering what matters most.

The female need to please

There are endless assumptions about women and the ways we should conduct our lives. We are hard-wired to be people pleasers and not to rock the boat or upset anyone. It's not deemed lady-like to be angry, and much of the anger that can arise in our forties is not just hormonal, but also the result of keeping a lid on things for too long. Keeping our real feelings and needs to ourselves is exhausting, and by the time I got to my mid-forties I was finding it a challenge to get through the day without screaming. This anger was often misdirected and would result in me hurling stuff out of windows or breaking stuff. I even once set fire to my daughter's lunch box and half-terrified her to death (I apologised, of course). Now I look back on it, I was feeling the cumulative tension of years of saying, 'Oh no, I'm fine, I don't need a drink, thanks', or 'I agree with what David just said about the brand strategy', or 'Does anyone want a top-up of tea?' Despite being raised by a feminist family, I felt my needs should always be placed at the bottom of the pile. I'd absorbed the wider social discourse instead. I noticed that if I was too loud or outspoken, then somebody would critique me and cut me down. I saw that in meetings if I got the courage to say something, I'd be immediately attacked (often by women more senior than me), so I became scared and didn't say anything. I feel frustrated when I think of how much time at work I wasted, listening to men drone on – usually re-jigging something they'd read in a clever book and passing it off as their own thinking. I would just sit there and be seething inside but didn't have the guts to argue with them because I wanted to be liked. I wanted to please. I wanted to be nice. Well, one thing I've learnt is that being nice only gets you so far and it's actually incredibly bad for you. The headaches, stomach complaints, insomnia I suffered from being nice were the serious side effects of not speaking up or upsetting anyone. On my way home from work I would listen to angry music – usually Courtney Love or Brody Dalle – and imagine I was an ultra-assertive, confident rock front woman. The reality couldn't have been further from the truth. I still managed to get to the top of the tree, but if you'd asked my colleagues to describe me, they'd have said something like: 'Oh yeah… Anniki. She's the nice one. She's so sweet.'

One of the benefits of ageing is that the desire to please wears off. This is why so many older women are seen as grumpy. They're not – they've just stopped saying insipid things.

I spoke to Meg Mathews recently and it seems that finally there is a new definition of ageing – one that is more truthful and honest about the challenges of ageing rather than trying to pretend things are hunky dory when they're not.

> I hate the word 'role models', but for me, the women I look up to are everyday women that share and talk about their journeys. The women who are taking the challenge of ageing on and coming out the other side. Those women are brave because they're connecting and talking truthfully about what's happening.

The *people pleasing* can of course continue in our forties and fifties, but I've found that I tend to be more aware when I'm doing it and less prepared to keep it up for very long. A good indication that your relationship with someone is genuine is if you are truly saying what you think and not holding back, worried about whether they'll judge you or not. If you are worried, then they're probably not right for you anyway.

The middle way – how to cope with ageing in a way that works for you (and is not defined by others' expectations)

Is there a middle way then when it comes to ageing? A way that is not middle-aged? A way that doesn't demand that we keep on going at the same pace and intensity as we did in our thirties but also doesn't expect us to calm down and sport comfy slacks either? So, some way of ageing that feels slightly more relaxing and won't lead to mental health problems, exhaustion and resentment?

I think there *is* a way to navigate through ageing, and this book will tell you how. Through a combination of interviews with women experiencing the ageing process and experts, research, and my personal experience of trying to re-invent myself in my late forties, it will show you how to not give up when ageing creeps up, and how to find a positive middle way that doesn't make you feel middle-aged. It will show you that it's okay to still be ambitious; there's no need to retire into cardigans and comfy slacks just yet. It will also show you how liberating it is to let go of all the unnecessary things *that no longer serve you*, as the yoga teachers of the world say.

There IS hope.

CHAPTER TWO

Why It's Okay to Do Something to Your Face, but Don't Do Too Much, Okay?

The Day I Decided to Do Something

I picked up my phone on a whim during a particularly taxing day at work. I dialled the number I'd seen on my Instagram feed. The doctor picked up right away (she WAS a doctor and I felt that this was a good sign because I'd read that injectables weren't highly regulated and anyone could inject stuff into your face, if they fancied it).

'So tell me,' she said, after we'd done the initial pleasantries about the weather/fact she was based near where I'd grown up in south London, 'what's bothering you? What would you like to improve about your appearance?'

I considered her question for a moment. 'I look tired,' I said. 'Even after a good night's sleep, I look knackered. I have lines on either side of my mouth that makes me look depressed, like a Basset Hound.'

'Yes, go on,' the doctor said encouragingly.

I could feel myself warming to the subject now. 'My eyes are shrinking. I have this frown line which means I look grumpy. And sometimes I *am* grumpy. I mean I'm forty-three and have a three-year-old who doesn't sleep through the night but I want to look like there's still some life in this old dog.'

'Do you want to come in and we can do a consultation?' she said. 'We can discuss things in more detail then.'

I hung up. I felt like I was doing something positive. Maybe some of you are reading this and thinking, 'YOU TRAITOR! YOU ARE JUST SUBSCRIBING TO THE MALE VISION OF WHAT WOMEN SHOULD LOOK LIKE. YOU SHOULD BE WRINKLED AND HAPPY.' Yes, I will come to this later, but the truth is I was just sick of looking tired. If the female vision of what women should look like was one of looking tired, then I didn't hold much truck with it anymore.

A week later, I arrived at the clinic, my heart thundering in my chest at the thought of what I was about to do (I am a feminist after all) but also excited that perhaps there was a way to feel better about how my face was looking these days. Besides, why shouldn't I do this? I say this even though at the time I felt like I should have a wig on and a headscarf just in case I saw any other feminists and they'd judge me. In my head I carried this little two-voice narrative. The first voice was my step-mum who was an ardent feminist.

> **Voice one:** *What the fuck are you doing, you empty headed dolt?*
>
> **Voice two:** *Listen, I have a good job. I work bloody hard. I deserve to pamper myself, right?*
>
> **Voice one:** *But this isn't pampering! You're lying to yourself. You're basically going to pay someone to inject poison into your face. You went to Greenham Common as a child!*
>
> **Voice two:** *Listen, everyone's doing it. Nobody is admitting to it though. Have you watched* Big Little Lies? *Do you think those actors really look that way from fresh air and exercise? What about that weird hair that started growing out of your boob? Did you just leave it to grow two feet long? Is that what natural beauty means to you?*

> **Voice one:** *It's not the same thing at all. I'm seriously disappointed. You read* The Beauty Myth. *You might not remember all the content but you did, right?*
>
> **Voice two:** *Yes, I read it. Yes, I remember some of it, but why shouldn't I be allowed to do what I want with my face?*

Sadly, my step-mum died three decades ago under very tragic circumstances, and the truth is that feminism back then had a certain set of expectations around what women should look like. When we went to Greenham common, all the women had short hair. It was a rejection of the patriarchal order and it was cool. My step-mum also wore no make-up, had hairy legs and armpits, and often wore a boilersuit. She'd have thought I was selling out, succumbing to the traditional definitions of what makes women attractive, like having a juicy, glowing face. She used to call people 'plastic' if they wore too much make-up. The older I became, the more I became consumed by my looks: I permed my hair, wore mini-skirts, shaved my eyebrows off, shaved just about all my hair off; I rebelled against some of the more restrictive dictates.

Growing up, I'd laughed like every other woman when I saw someone who'd had terrible cosmetic surgery. There were lots of examples as many celebrities tried things out for the first time and got it wrong. In my early thirties I knew I'd never be one of those poor saps that chased the fountain of youth. Besides, it was undignified to do that all the time, right? I changed my mind as soon as I hit my mid-forties and woke up each morning looking like I'd had no sleep, drunk a litre of vodka and smoked forty fags.

In an ideal world the way we look wouldn't matter, but the truth is it does

In the future we may all be avatars that we've designed ourselves and we will hover about in the air and be half-butterfly and half-Danish pastry with Goldie Hawn's head stuck on top. But right now, in this particular time, looks matter. They always have done. We look at someone and make a bunch of assumptions about them based on what they're wearing, how frizzy their hair is, whether they have tattoos or not (I'm tattooed and still get people judging me and assuming that I also drink Jack Daniels and smoke roll-ups). Aged forty-three I'd also found myself competing at work with women half my age. I knew that when I went into a meeting and looked exhausted, it didn't help my cause. This sounds superficial and daft perhaps, but haven't you found yourself doing the same thing with people around you?

For me it wasn't about looking old and trying to run away from that because I wanted to be twenty-three again. Instead, it was the fact that I still looked like dog shit even after a rare good night of sleep. There are times when you walk into a room to do a presentation and the first thing people will think is 'Jeez, she looks fucking knackered,' and that can get in the way of your communication skills – even if you've brushed your hair and put on a decent top. It basically means people won't listen to you. Of course, there are exceptions, but in the industry I worked in at that time (communications and marketing), women were youthful and fashionably dressed. I'd been in board meetings where a male director had gone through the female CVs, looking at photos and putting them into two piles: 'I'd fuck them' and 'I'd not touch them with a barge pole'. This culture was rife and resulted in a company of beautiful women (many of them super bright, too) and not-so-attractive men (the male directors perhaps not wanting to hire males that might provide visual competition). Of course, I didn't respect this culture, but I also knew on a rational level that certain visual traits got in the way of how you were perceived at work. I'd been distracted by a male colleague who had yellow tombstone teeth. I hoped that looking less tired would help me stay in the game (I wasn't bothered whether any of the directors wanted to sleep with me or not) and would also make me feel more confident after coming back from maternity leave to discover that my role had been changed and I was now being bossed about by people I'd hired twelve months previously.

You may still be shouting at me that I should have tackled my position at work and the industry I worked in instead of getting Botox, and you're right. On reflection, I could have done more to try and change things. And I should have done so, too.

But I had wrinkles and I didn't like them on my face.

Back at the clinic, the doctor showed me some examples of work she had done on other patients. We then had a quick discussion and I very quickly decided to go ahead with her suggestions.

'I'll be doing injections here and here,' she said, holding up a mirror so I could see where she was pointing – just to the side of each eye and the space between my eyebrows. 'And then we will do a bit of filler here and here,' she said, pointing at a space near my cheekbone and another near my mouth.

I nodded.

'There is something called "the golden ratio" that is associated with the ideal definition of beauty. We can do certain measurements and we find all the classically beautiful faces share this ratio.'

My heart was really going off now and I felt like I was about to take heroin or have an affair with a married man. The first voice was screeching in my ears, 'WHAT ARE YOU DOING? WHAT IF YOU END UP LOOKING LIKE CHER? ARE YOU GOING TO WORK ON MONDAY LOOKING LIKE CHER? EVERYONE WILL LAUGH THEIR HEAD OFF! AND WHAT ON EARTH WOULD YOUR STEP-MUM THINK?'

'So, are you sure you're happy to go ahead?' she asked.

I nodded. I have a dangerous habit of agreeing to things when every cell in my body is telling me it's a mistake. This is also why I have a giant tattoo on one forearm that is five times larger than I intended, and a design that I really wasn't sure about but went ahead with it anyway as I was too intimidated to tell the visiting tattoo artist from New Orleans that I wanted something smaller and more girly.

'Have you had any work done on yourself?' I asked the doctor.

She didn't have any lines. Even when she was examining me, her face remained remarkably flat and expressionless. 'Not yet, but I will eventually. You won't regret it,' she said. 'Right, now lie back and there will be a short wait whilst I get everything ready.'

I could have told her to get stuffed with her speech about the ideal beauty ratio bollocks and told her I was happy as I was. I could have said that I was happy to be ignored. I could have told her I didn't care that I looked seriously knackered all the time or that I was obsessed with looking at celebrities' faces and trying to see what they'd done to look so excellent. Instead, I lay there, my heart pounding, feeling like I was being unfaithful to myself, my sisterhood and my step-mum, and worried that I was going to look weird. I imagined myself with a giant balloon face and everyone laughing, and having to go on talk shows to explain my own awful vanity.

That wasn't what happened at all.

Half an hour later I emerged from the clinic and went to meet my best friend for a coffee. A quick note on my friend Amy, who is mentioned several times in this book. She is not my ONLY FRIEND but she is someone I have known since I was eleven and even though we don't see one another regularly, we have shared a lot of 'key moments' together. She is also the same age as me, so has been consistent throughout my life. Amy has basically been the one who has held my hair back when I've retched into a toilet in a nightclub. We've slept in the same bed, bathed together, cried together. We argued in the past because I discovered her diary and it said how much she hated me (like all teenage friendships we had our ups and downs). One thing you need to know about Amy is she is *beautiful*. And was a model. And I spent much of my adolescence standing in clubs in the West End with men approaching me only because they wanted to go out with her, which is perhaps why I found myself getting the FULL WORKS at the clinic thirty-odd years later. The truth was I'd always felt ugly. I'd been plagued with a poor body image and had fantasised that I'd follow Amy into modelling (I was pretty but had short fat legs like a rugby player, so it was never going to happen).

'So, what did you have done, you dingbat?' she said. 'You are silly. I mean I get it, but how much did it cost and won't you have to keep going back to have more stuff done?'

'Well,' I said, 'I got some Botox injections and this filler stuff in my cheeks.'

'I can't see any difference,' she said, studying my face intently.

I was sitting in the sun and my skin felt a bit uncomfortable, but my face hadn't exploded. I didn't look like I'd been stretched out in the sun. In fact, I looked pretty much the same. I was actually disappointed that there wasn't a more noticeable difference right away.

'It'll take a few days apparently.'

'I'm not judging. It's your face.'

'You will tell me if I look weird though, right?' I said nervously. On the tube on the way home the internal narrative continued.

> **Voice one:** *You stupid fool. You're going to look like a right weirdo. I've got a direct line to your step-mum and she is seriously pissed.*
> **Voice two:** *It's nothing to be ashamed of. Look, there's actually no difference. It's not like I've got my head stuck in a wind tunnel!*
> **Voice one:** *You've just paid a few hundred quid to have a stranger inject chemicals into your face.*
> **Voice two:** *Times change. It's 2017. Look at the flipping Kardashians – they've built a whole career on looking a certain way!*
> **Voice one:** *So, you want to be a Kardashian? Jeez. You really are a deluded fool, woman. You disappoint me. You can't even remember who you are.*

Voice two: *Be quiet. I just want to feel like my life isn't over. I just want to look less fucking tired!*

About ten days passed. Ten days with no noticeable side effects, bar a small bruise on the side of my head that was easily covered with concealer. No feminists came knocking on my door. I wasn't struck down by a bolt of lightning bursting out of the hand of an angry female goddess.

I just looked less tired.

When you look tired even when you're not tired

Ageing isn't necessarily about the avoidance of looking old but is sometimes more about our faces no longer reflecting the way we feel. I often used to think my boss was grumpy, and she probably was grumpy having to fight the patriarchy all day but she also lost the ability to convey any other kind of emotion aside from extreme grumpiness, even if she'd just won a big client account and had a glass of prosecco in her hand. So, some of us end up with our face less able to convey our mood and we may like to pretend that it doesn't matter, but in some industries and contexts it does. This doesn't mean you have to rush to get Botox but it does mean acknowledging the current reality and whether you're up for going against the tide, which is courageous and noble but also (for me anyway) hard work on top of everything else.

For me, it's more about ME FEELING LIKE I'm still part of the cut and thrust, feeling relevant, feeling alive.

'What skin cream have you been using?' a colleague asked a couple of months after the visit to the clinic. 'You look great.'

I hesitated for a moment. Should I tell her the truth? I decided not to. I knew I'd be judged. I'd judged other women too. I would have to pretend like everyone else did.

'Oh, I've just been getting a bit more sleep.'

'Well, I wish I looked like that with more sleep.'

I'd spent my entire life buying serums and creams and massaging my face and trying out different facials, but this thing worked. Despite the fact that I was perfectly happy with what I'd done and had managed to drown out VOICE NUMBER ONE, I still felt like I couldn't be open and honest about having tried injectables. I still felt a sense of shame. Shame that I was vain, that I'd given into the pressure to look a certain way. And this perception – the idea that women who have tweakments are superficial, stupid and vain – persists.

Why don't more women talk about Botox and injectables?

In my small online survey of 370 women aged 30–50 years, there was a sentiment that cosmeceuticals are becoming more acceptable. Fifty-three per cent agreed that they'd like to try them or are thinking about having them in the future. The cosmetic surgery industry is now worth £3.6 billion in the UK, with non-surgical treatments like Botox and fillers accounting for nine out of ten procedures and worth £2.75 billion.

Despite the rising popularity of injectables, the media tends to dismantle women who have work done on themselves and at the same time ridicules those women who don't. It uses adjectives like 'haggard', 'stressed' and 'worn out' when showing close-ups of older celebrities who haven't had work, and then underlines how 'smooth,' 'glowing' and 'youthful' they are if they have had something done.

Sali Hughes explained a bit more about this ambivalent relationship the media has with women and ageing:

> There seems to be a sweet spot where the press will allow you to exist without comment – a narrow range of WOMEN who have

had work done but not in an obvious way – THEN the press will still be nice about you so you're getting away with it being 'natural'. Someone has to PASS FOR 'naturally beautiful' or they don't pass muster.

The whole area is rife with contradictions. This instils fear into some women – fear that they will be judged as silly and vain or bird-brained. (The younger generation doesn't necessarily share these fears as they've grown up against a different backdrop. They have different pressures though.) On a personal level, I've always been pissed off when I read another interview with a woman in her forties or fifties and there is no mention of the fact that she's done anything to her face besides having nice early nights and rubbing pineapple on her brow. I feel like it isn't honest; like they're leading us down the garden path, despite the fact that I've not been honest about having work done on my face either.

Sali has a very different perspective on why we shouldn't press women on whether they've had work done:

> I don't know why women should be held accountable for how they look. We don't hold men accountable in the same way, do we? And must that woman also declare what serum she's used or whether she's dyed her hair? How much does this woman have to bare her soul to you?

When she said this, I knew I was doing the very thing that the mainstream media/society-at-large was doing – looking at older women and judging whether I was happy with the way they'd chosen to age. I was no better than the *Daily Mail*'s sidebar of shame.

One issue, however, with nobody admitting to having cosmeceutical work is that there is less information out there on the reputable places to go and which ones to avoid, how much you should think of paying for a treatment, what might go wrong and how to choose the right person. If we all pretend that we're not doing it, then none of this information goes out into the public domain. Part of the reason I wanted to talk to Sali was because she has spoken out on the subject and has been so open and honest about the tweakments she's undertaken. I'd found this refreshing and interesting. But what about feminism? Sali sees no conflict here:

> My mum was a strident feminist and was very politically engaged, but I didn't have a dictate about my appearance or how I should look. I am allergic to statements like 'women should' or 'feminists should' – if one isn't applying the same rules to a man, then it's sexist.

It's true that dictating what is right and what is wrong when it comes to women's appearance and ageing isn't right either. It comes back to the point that women should be able to choose. And in order to choose, we need to be more honest about what we're doing with our faces and not pretend it's just smoothies or a good sex life.

It's also about being well-rounded humans. In the classic book *The Beauty Myth*, Naomi Wolf explains how modern women have effectively become beauty, whereas in previous generations, women would have become their ovaries. So, beauty becomes the only thing we are recognised for nowadays. (You could argue our ovaries are also valued and are constantly discussed in terms of how fertile we are, when we're going to reproduce, whether we're going to reproduce, what age that's going to happen, etc.)

The fact that I've had Botox in the past doesn't define the kind of person I am. I am a woman who sometimes has Botox but is also raising two daughters as feminists. I believe women and men should share the domestic load. I want to be paid as much as my male colleagues. I don't worship at the altar of consumerism. (Well, if it's a jumpsuit, then I do, but I am also trying to be more conscious of what I buy and whether I need it and where it comes from.) I also believe that I can care about the way I look AND be more than just the way I look, so that I can read difficult books, do an *Arrow* word puzzle and have a fairly well-informed conversation about Brexit.

I would never bully another woman into getting Botox and I'm not saying every woman should do it. I *will* say that it made me look less tired and this made me feel better.

When I interviewed Meg Mathews (who has been open about the treatments she's had done), she acknowledged that there is more openness now; and if women choose to be frank and honest about it, then there is possibly less judgement – there is nothing to 'reveal' if it's already been talked about, and we can all move on and talk about other important stuff like the menopause, the gender pay gap, race inequality, domestic violence and the motherload. Meg said:

> Ten years ago I wouldn't have said I'd had fillers because then the press would have been scathing about it. Now I speak my truth because I've already said it so the media don't come out about it. They have written awful things in the past. I want to share with women because what I do doesn't cost millions of pounds and it is fairly accessible too.

What is this 'ageing naturally' thing anyway?

When you're twenty, you can possibly walk around in a white shirt and a pair of pants (I was never one of those women), wear no make-up and have unbrushed hair and be like a sexy, interesting, attractive person. But I've discovered that none of us are NATURAL in our approach to beauty. Do you pull an errant nose hair out with tweezers? Well, that's not natural. Do you dye your roots? Do you squeeze a pimple? What does 'natural' actually mean? If I truly allowed myself to age naturally, I would have the following attributes and facial characteristics:

- a white beard
- purple bags under my eyes
- the odd random long eyebrow that sticks out and gets in the way of my right eye.

These are just some of the things that I choose to hide from the world at large. It would be preferable if we lived in a world where white beards and hairy noses didn't get in the way of how people perceived you, but THEY DO. I'm also not sure I want to be the trailblazer in terms of championing my beard (which is hereditary and has only really taken off in my forties). I want to be able to write and talk at events, and do podcasts and interviews, and not be seen as the woman who looks like Kris Kristofferson. If this makes me superficial and stupid, then so be it. I also don't see me caring about having a beard as being incompatible with caring about how women aren't paid as much as men or face harassment at work or have to do all the domestic and emotional labour.

Many women in my survey felt conflicted by things like injectables. They were mourning their changing faces but also felt worried and nervous about taking any 'radical' steps. Here are some of the things they said:

I look in the mirror and just feel really depressed.

I don't recognise myself anymore.

I don't think my face reflects who I am. I am only forty-one but look ten years older than that.

I hate the fact that I look so tired and everything looks weary and saggy, but I don't want to look strange either.

It's an individual choice, but we need to stop pretending that nobody is doing it and the people who are doing it are weird or that only weird-looking people do it in the first place.

Okay, but isn't this stuff addictive? Don't you start off doing one thing and then end up with loads of stuff done?

I would say that, yes, it is possible to get addicted to the results of cosmetic work. And it's very important to choose a practitioner who is not going to take advantage of your insecurities. The other thing to consider – and this is a biggie – is the expense involved. If you're like me and think the results are worth it, then you may want to carry on investing in it. Sometimes they say you need to either choose your body or your face and I've opted for my face. This does make taking my clothes off rather alarming as there is a definite difference between face and body. (I don't think there is a show yet called *How Old Does My Body Look?*, where you stand naked in the street, but if there were such a programme, I would easily look ten years older than I really am.)

My bikini line is out of order, my cellulite is all over the place and I have an odd, blobby tummy that hasn't gone back to normal after having children. I don't feel like I'm under the same kind of pressure as other women, and I pick and choose what I care about and what matters less appearance-wise. I'm not a celebrity who has an unlimited budget and is under immense pressure because I'm going to be papped whilst on holiday in Mykonos. I don't have to see myself on the cover of a magazine with big neon circles drawing attention to my boobs and an accompanying caption that reads 'Sad, saggy, boobs drive X to drink'. I think we need to better understand why so many female celebrities push the envelope surgery-wise – it's because we put them under a microscope and interrogate their flaws. It is because of misogyny. It is because we are taught to hate our appearance from a young age.

One thing I'm not sure about is whether I will continue to have Botox. I've not had it for a while now and don't want to feel dependent on it. Truth be told, I can't really afford to keep paying for it. I don't have the cash and don't feel it's appropriate to start a crowdfunding page to help my flabby jaws. And whilst I talk about a middle way, a new definition of ageing, I sometimes feel nostalgic for the days when women could put on their camel-coloured cardigans and tartan slippers and have Yorkshire Terriers called Mufty and spend their days eating shortbread.

Also, it's perfectly fine if you choose not to have work done. Using sun cream, good make-up, investing in a night cream, a healthy diet, sleep – all these things will help your skin look its best – *but*, let's get rid of the shame and guilt around wanting to look less tired and let's stop penalising women for taking action if they're happy enough to do so. Let's not tell women how to age and let's allow them to decide for themselves. Also, let's be honest with others if we have had work done. It's not about interrogating women and outing them; *rather*, it's more authentic to tell people so they can make an informed decision if they decide to go down that route.

Here are some useful tips from Sali Hughes if you are thinking of getting something done:

- Always aim to see a doctor rather than a nurse or beauty therapist.
- Ensure you really trust the person who is treating you and have a good rapport.

- Word of mouth is important. If you have a friend and like what they've had done and think it's a good job, and the doctor comes recommended, then that's a good sign.
- Be wary of a doctor who tries to add to your wish list. A good doctor should ask you what you see as being the problem but shouldn't be trying to sell you more stuff you don't need. If they are telling you that you don't need certain tweakments, then that's a good sign.
- Make sure that the person you're meeting for your consultation is the same person who will be doing your tweakment. Lots of clinics use sales people as the first port of call, but you need to insist that you see the person who will be treating you.
- Let things wear off before going back for more – this way you can keep an eye on things and don't risk losing perspective on what's normal.

And from my own perspective, I would say don't get Botox or injectables because it's something you feel you SHOULD do. Or feel bullied into it. BULLY BOTOX is never a good idea.

One of the quotes from my survey which really struck me was this:

I feel like I never really got a chance to be comfortable with who I am, how I look. When I was younger, I hated the way I looked, and now I'm getting older I still hate the way I look, but with the addition of wrinkles.

Ultimately, as women there will always be a set of expectations from ourselves and society at large in terms of how we should look. We can acknowledge and accept certain things about our appearance and that's okay, but we can also be aware that there are options if we want them, whether those options are using nice face creams or going to get some Botox.

For many of us, the sense that we don't look good enough is something that's followed us around all our lives. There is something to be said for giving yourself some real and pragmatic self-talk. It's a strange time because it feels like injectables won't be so much of a taboo in the future (already they're not for many younger women) and then there will be more of a conversation around them – both generally and more honestly. The thing is, if you do opt to try them, it doesn't mean you've signed an agreement that says you will continue to do it for the rest of your life. It's like dying your hair rose-gold. If you don't like it, then you just don't do it again. Nobody is standing over you with a giant needle and forcing it into your forehead (or if they are, then they're not a good person and you need to run away because nobody should be forcing Botox into your face against your will).

Whatever your approach to ageing and beauty, it's important to not let it dominate your life. It doesn't make you superficial or stupid to care about it in the first place and it doesn't define you – not unless you let it. This is what I tell myself anyway. There are far more important things to focus on – like finding work that inspires you, building good relationships with your friends and not letting life grind you down when the going gets tough.

Four reasons not to worry too much about what you look like

1. No one cares.
2. No one notices.
3. No one cares.
4. No one notices.

This was a big revelation. I have now realised, in my late forties, that people may comment on a nice, floral blouse you're wearing, or a new pair of trainers, but they don't notice much else. They don't notice whether you've washed your hair, or whether you have primer on, or even the fact that you may have a few stray chin hairs. I know this is true as I don't notice THE DETAILS of people and their appearance either. I don't get a magnifying glass out and check to see whether they have applied serum first and then primer and then foundation. I don't notice if they've got no make-up on. Or if their roots are growing through. Women's magazines talk to us as if these tiny details, such as having nice nails, or pumicing the dead skin off our feet or exfoliating our pores, are the most important things in life. If I read one more article about 'dry skin body brushing' and how it combats cellulite, I will drop dead.

I love looking after myself and I want to feel good when I look in the mirror, but I don't expect other people to applaud because I've shaved my legs or managed to do the 'perfect black liner' on my eyes.

Do these things for yourself but for nobody else (unless your chin is really hairy like mine, and then people definitely notice and are appalled and frightened and actively avoid talking to you).

This is important to remember. The main person who notices what's going on with your appearance is YOU. Everyone else is too worried about their own personal flaws to get hung up on yours.

Ten things to do before turning fifty

1. **Do some outdoor river/lake swimming:** I keep seeing people doing this and want to give it a go myself. Apparently it improves your circulation, boosts your immunity and helps you sleep. I suspect I won't like it because I don't like green, slimey stuff on my feet or the idea that there are fish with teeth nibbling at my toes.

2. **Drive the car on a motorway:** I passed my test two years ago but have become one of those people who never drives so am now terrified of the idea of being on a motorway. In fact, at the moment I won't even drive to the supermarket, so perhaps I need to do that first and then progress to the motorway.

3. **Visit Big Sur in California and stay in one of the log cabins deep in the redwood forest:** We did a trip to California years ago, but the cabin we stayed in was right next to the main road so wasn't quite as idyllic as it should have been.

4. **Crowd surf:** I'm not sure how realistic this is, what with Covid-19 and the fact that I'm pushing thirteen stone right now and few people will want to raise me above their head for fear of being squashed to death.

5. **Smoke a doobie:** I haven't smoked spliff for many years but I'm thinking that post-fifty I might take it up properly and have a small joint once a week in the garden as a Friday treat (or in the local park with the other mums as an alternative to talking about sports day/house prices/local café being too expensive, etc.)

6. **Write a TV adaptation with Sharon Horgan:** I've been putting this 'out there' for some time and mention it again here in case Sharon is reading this and wants someone to collaborate with. I sense she possibly has a lot of people who want to work with her, but does she have a crowd-surfing, spliff-smoking, motorway-driving fifty-something? Doubt it.

7. **Tell someone I hate to FUCK OFF:** I have never told anyone to fuck off in my entire life (apart from a partner and that doesn't count does it?). Even people that have got right up in my face and irritated the hell out of me. I want to know what it feels like to really shout it out and feel the release rather than bottling it up and walking away and muttering it under my breath, then bitching about that person behind their back. I imagine this will be the BEST FEELING EVER.

8. **Go skinny dipping:** Maybe in the river, maybe with a doobie – so combining number 1, 5 and 8 together.

9. **Get another tattoo:** Yes, I know, classic midlife crisis, but I have a big space on my forearm that's ripe for another one and this time I am really GOING FOR IT.

10. **Go to Glastonbury:** I'm sick of listening to people describe it as 'life changing' and 'a real spiritual awakening'. I want to experience it first-hand, without children, without my partner – ideally with a bunch of female friends. I want to see everything there is to see instead of sitting on the sofa, watching it on TV, with a flavoured cider and a packet of Doritos. I want to finally wear the kind of outfit Jo Whiley wears – something like a glittery cape with sequins, and maybe even a wig. I don't even care if teenagers take photos of me and snigger behind my back because I look fucking ridiculous.

CHAPTER THREE

Ageing, Infertility and Motherhood – It's a Real Ball Ache

How Sex Education Never Teaches Us about Infertility

When I was at school the main point of sex education seemed to be instructing you on how to avoid pregnancy. Oh, and how to put a condom on a banana. I remember becoming hysterical the first time I slept with a boy (I don't think his penis had successfully entered me but he'd ejaculated somewhere on my thigh because my wet-look perm and frosted Boots 17 bronze lipstick had fired him up like an ejaculating Catherine wheel).

'I need the morning-after pill,' I said to Amy the following day.

We were sat on the beach. We were in Spain. We went to the same place in Spain every year because Amy's parents had a small holiday house there. Let's just say that we did a lot of very silly things, like many teenagers growing up at that time did (this was before parents followed you around with their phone and asked you to text every three minutes). On this particular morning I was full of remorse and had peeling shoulders and a light hangover (remember when hangovers passed after a couple of hours instead of going on for days?).

'What do you mean? You didn't have sex with him, did you? You know he's a gigolo, right?' Amy said with disdain. 'Don't you remember his friend told us he was a sex worker?' (This wasn't true. Or if it was, then he wasn't a skilled gigolo as the sex had been terrible. Not that we'd had sex – not that I could remember anyway.)

The 'gigolo' I'd had clumsy, awful 'sex' with also had a wet-look perm. It must have been the 'hot-wet-look-perm summer of '88'. I'd said the words 'NO BABIES' in his ear whilst he was writhing about on top of me (I've never been particularly good at talking dirty). I had no idea how to get a man to stop writhing about on top of you when you had no interest in them. It took me a few more years to understand that I didn't have to go with the flow, even if the refusal ran the risk of peeving men off, which is a lesson I want to get instilled in my daughters early on: YOU DO NOT HAVE TO SLEEP WITH A MAN BECAUSE YOU'RE WORRIED THAT IF YOU REFUSE, THINGS WILL FEEL WEIRD. The idea of being sixteen with a baby was terrifying. At this point in my life, I felt like there was a world of opportunity ahead – it was all vague and misty, but I was sure I was going to be a famous. I'd be doing something that involved working in the music industry, meeting pop stars, wearing a lot of expensive clothes, and driving a silver VW Beetle. Most of my ambitions were gleaned from watching TV adverts for sanitary towels and Impulse deodorant spray.

'Where on earth are we going to get the morning-after pill from?' Amy said, rubbing factor zero carrot oil on her legs (she was very fair, but these were the times when we didn't know about the harmful effects of UV light and still believed you had to burn before you could get a good tan). 'I don't think they hand them out to any old slags [we were avid readers of *Viz* magazine and liked the characters of the 'Two Fat Slags', so we used the term affectionately for one another] and I'm guessing you don't want to tell my parents and then have them call your parents.'

'Maybe I'll be okay,' I said, trying to think about what exactly had happened, not being completely convinced that his penis had actually gone anywhere near my vagina. I'd felt pain, though (this was only my second time with a boy, and the first time had also been a disaster for a myriad of reasons).

Was I pregnant?

Over the next few evenings, I'd sit and think about my baby. How I'd have to give up school. How it would have a perm. How it would never know its father. How I suspected the father was in fact a gigolo and travelled far and wide inflicting mediocre sex on poor girls who'd had too much vodka. I would have to bring the baby up on my own. I was too self-absorbed and had no mental band-width available to handle a child (I spent an inordinate amount of time worrying about the shape of my eyebrows and fantasising about either Ben from Curiosity or Michael Hutchence, or ideally both of them having a fight over me in a pub and me agreeing to go out with Ben first and then Michael later on).

It seems ironic that I was worried about getting pregnant by accident or that I thought it could happen so easily. It turned out that I wasn't pregnant and I breathed a sigh of relief. I started work, I became more responsible, I stopped going to Spain, I got a serious boyfriend and then another serious boyfriend and then I came off the pill when I was thirty-six and thought, 'Okay, now all my friends have kids and so I guess I better get moving because their kids aren't even babies anymore – they're like school age. And I'm not really sure why I'm sat in endless meetings talking about the future direction of fish fingers in Bulgaria [these were actual meetings that happened].'

You know that scene in *The Wizard of Oz* where Dorothy keeps tapping her red, sequined shoes together and chanting 'There's no place like home' over and over? That's how I anticipated getting pregnant would be. I knew it wasn't about tapping feet – that there was more INTIMACY required – but I really thought it would be super easy.

The bit where Anniki learns that some careers are not compatible with motherhood (unless you're so wealthy that you have one of those underground basement kitchens like Robbie Williams)

The desire to be a mum had somehow been shunted to the background because my career was really hard work. I worked in qualitative market research. (Don't worry, you probably haven't heard of it – it's basically doing a lot of talking to people in focus groups and getting them to buy stuff they don't want.) It involved long hours, lots of travel and evening work. The mums in the company didn't get to see their kids much and were dealing with a level of stress that I found hard to fathom – a juggling act that seemed impossible to maintain long term. There were senior women who had nannies, and these nannies seemed to be performing the role of super-efficient wife (I've always thought all successful women need a wife) – buying birthday gifts for kids' parties, ironing, ordering school uniforms and even filming school assemblies and editing them so the mums could watch them at more convenient times of the day (like before they got up at 6am to do tennis coaching or whatever it is that superwomen do). Even these BOSS women were prone to crying and anger, and I just couldn't visualise how I'd manage to have a kid and look after it and do the level of work I had (I was responsible at this time for doing about 90–100 appraisals, which felt like I was sitting in rooms having toxic emotional baggage thrown in my face over and over each and every day). I expected to magically find a new career somehow (without taking any action) and then it would be time to be a mother and my body would co-operate. I had zero awareness of fertility issues or treatment or how your fertility plunged off a sharp cliff once you hit thirty-five.

None of this had been shared in our sex ed lessons. I wish it had. I also wish they'd told me how to say no to sex with men I didn't like as this would have saved a lot of heartache.

Trying for a baby isn't fun

My partner and I started timing sex on certain days of the month. I was using these nifty ovulation kits which tell you the exact time you need to have sex to conceive. I was optimistic to start with. I got the kit. I had the sex. I expected the baby. After a year of doing this, I moved onto a more advanced digital ovulation kit which had a smiley face when you were ovulating. This made me feel more reassured that it was going to work – this idiotic smiley face. My friends' children were now getting older and my friends were telling me they were feeling so much better now they were 'out of the woods'. I was worried I was never going to get 'into the woods' at this stage. I was thirty-eight. The world of market research was pulling me into rounds of endless meetings and I'd been promoted to Managing Director. This meant more money but oodles of stress and politics to navigate. I became the 'peacemaker' – the one who essentially gets shit thrown in their face each day and has to shovel their way out of it. I found it harder to empathise with my colleagues. All I could see when I looked at them was a baby with goo goo eyes and chubby legs and an adorable curl at the front of its head.

'Oh, so you're worried that you've only been sent to Mexico this year and haven't done any other global strategic work,' you say. 'WELL, I WANT TO BE A MOTHER AND CANNOT GET PREGNANT AND AM STARTING TO PANIC! So, what do you say about that?'

When you want to get pregnant, all you notice is other pregnant women. They are like zombies coming out of the mist (only you don't want to shoot them, but maybe a part of you does because you feel so envious). Women younger than me got pregnant. I started to worry that there was something wrong with me. I started thinking about the fact that I'd NEVER fallen pregnant accidentally. My first boyfriend and I never even used contraception (we went through a bad patch where we stopped having sex and of course this was a very effective form of contraception, but even before that I'd never had a late period). My partner and I kept trying, which basically destroyed our love life (nobody tells you this either – you fully expect that you'll continue to want to have sex with one another even when it's become a chore), and then each month I'd feel my boobs getting achy and then my period would arrive, usually a few days late – just enough time to get my hopes up and then these hopes would be dashed.

'Selfish women who ran out of time'

I've read lots of media stories about women like me who have been deemed SELFISH because we put our careers first. I kind of wish I'd been more selfish and actively chosen a career and then been mistress of my own destiny, but the truth is life is what happens when you've got other plans (this isn't just a jaunty phrase on a novelty teacup). Right from the off I needed a job that paid money rather than one where you worked for free (my parents weren't loaded). I didn't have a clear idea of what career I wanted. Maybe this was my own fault because I spent too long day dreaming about a fake career in the music industry which involved no concrete work but mainly seducing rock singers and driving them around in my silver VW Beetle. It wasn't just the sex education at fault, it was the idea that you could have a career and a home and a family and everything would fall into place. We weren't schooled in thinking about our fertility and I didn't twig that having babies was something that needed to be thought about in advance if possible or that fertility was a finite commodity like water draining out of a leaky bucket.

When people say you can have it all, they are lying (this is one of the things that it has taken me forty-seven years to learn)

I'd never really felt connected with my body in any meaningful way. I knew there were eggs in there somewhere but didn't really make the connection with how they age just like the rest of us and that their quality isn't so great once you reach your late thirties. Nobody said that once you got to forty your chances of falling pregnant naturally were probably 5 per cent. Nobody said that you might not be able to have kids.

I had tests but there was nothing wrong. There doesn't have to be anything wrong. You start to realise that getting pregnant is really a miracle. My partner had tests too but there was nothing wrong there either. We were just old. I opted for fertility treatment. I was lucky because I had a well-paid job and savings. I realise that lots of women aren't in this position and have to get into massive debt or can't continue if the NHS round(s) don't work (and how many cycles you get is different depending on where you live).

'The man puts his penis into the woman's vagina and he thrusts, and then the semen comes out and this is how a baby is made,' Mrs Hill told me in sex education.

I had four cycles of in vitro fertilisation (IVF), three miscarriages and then finally got pregnant and had my daughter on the last round. I then had another two rounds and got pregnant with my second daughter (moving me into the Janet Jackson age of motherhood – almost). This history isn't that bad when it comes to fertility treatment. For a start, I did actually wind up with kids. I've had friends who've had ten rounds and failed to get pregnant. I also had a friend who was about to give up on having children and then got pregnant on her eleventh round. The thing is that it's very hard to throw in the towel. There's always a sense that success is around the corner; and if you have a failed round, then you want to keep going. One friend has remained childless and has gone on to have a fantastic life (because, newsflash, you can have a brilliant life without kids). But just to be clear, fertility treatment wears you down. It exhausts you. It makes you obsessive. It gives you blinkers. It makes you want to kick pregnant women up the arse. It makes you desperate. It makes you anxious.

It's a complex, dastardly beast and wonderful at the same time (if it works that is).

The reality of going through fertility treatment

One of the clinics I went to had a punishing regime where you had to arrive every morning at 7am to have your blood tested. This meant getting up at 5am, taking the tube into town, queuing with a bunch of worried, anxious women (most of us so worried that we didn't really speak to each other) and then heading into work, pretending everything was normal and trying to be a useful professional whilst crying in the toilet at regular intervals. I didn't want people at work to know I was having treatment. I was worried that they'd ask me about it. I was also worried that it would compromise my position as the women who had babies were generally viewed as below par. (There was a definite sense that once you had a child, unless you were a machine, you weren't as good at your job as you'd been beforehand.)

In the second week of treatment, you had to hang around the clinic and wait for a phone call. Once the call came, you were told exactly how much stimulating hormone you needed to inject yourself with, and I got very adept at finding clean toilets. I usually opted for John Lewis, next to the baby department, which made the injecting experience more poignant as I brushed past the teddies and breast pumps on my way there and back, hoping that soon I'd be browsing these things because I'd actually BE PREGNANT – please, please, please, God.

And miscarriages. Unfortunately, they seemed to be fairly common. My eggs just weren't up to scratch, or the moon wasn't in Cancer, or perhaps it was my blood, or it was the fact that I'd ACTUALLY LEFT MOTHERHOOD A LITTLE TOO LATE BUT HADN'T GOT THE MEMO. The second pregnancy went wrong at eleven weeks. We were just due to have the first scan after the weekend. I woke in the night with severe cramps – it felt like someone was twisting me inside out and I rushed straight to the toilet. I felt a WHOOSH down below and everything fell out. I say *everything*, but of course it was the baby. When we got to hospital, they kept asking me if they could test the 'material' to see what had happened, but it had all gone down the toilet.

The language is strange. When you have a scan and everything is okay, then it's a 'baby'. When you have a scan and it's gone wrong it's 'material that needs removing'.

There have thankfully only been a couple of times that I've cried like I did after that miscarriage. I kept thinking not only about the baby and the fact that I was no longer pregnant but also about all the early mornings, the injections, the smoothies, the vitamins, the crouching down in John Lewis's toilets squinting at little glass vials, trying to work out what I needed to do next, the way I'd always pick up little beanie hats and then put them down because I knew it was bad luck to buy anything for a baby before it arrived, but surely this time I was due a lucky break? Surely this was my time to be a mum? Sadly, no, it wasn't. And it can all disappear so quickly.

The paramedics were men and they were nice but they stood at the bottom of my bed like a couple of bouncers standing outside a cheesy nightclub in Leicester Square (they gathered themselves eventually but I think they were unsure of the best approach because I was howling and incoherent). Nothing would calm me down. I was having this strange conversation where I questioned myself and then provided the answer: 'Has the baby gone?' and then 'No, it can't have gone,' and then 'Yes it has gone,' and then 'No, it can't have gone'. I was worried that perhaps they'd put me in a straitjacket, but then there was something soothing about being put in a straitjacket, maybe even ushered into a padded cell, and then being given a massive amount of valium and just being comatose. A cell with soft walls and lots of drugs and maybe not having to wake up for a few weeks – these are things that you long for in desperate times – just to stop time completely. Maybe some Sigur Ros playing in the background too. There are times when you don't want to face reality – you just long for oblivion.

The thing is there wasn't any good news to wake up to, so I just wanted to sleep for as long as possible. At home I received lots of flower deliveries and I mooched about like a ghost in my ugly, towelling dressing gown and tried not to think about the bath I'd had when I'd got home, and how I'd found something in the bath which looked like part of my baby.

I took vitamins. I did acupuncture. I kept my head down. I saw babies everywhere. I grew incredibly superstitious and started to carry various lucky charms with me. I rubbed a rosary every night. I slept with my fingers crossed. I rubbed a Buddha each time I passed it beside the window pane. I touched my temple when I saw a single magpie. I only chewed food on one side of my mouth. I didn't step on cracks in the pavement. I lit candles whenever I was in a church. I was living in this magical, witchy time where everything I did was geared towards getting pregnant.

'Your levels are really high and you've got a strong pregnancy.'

It was New Year's Eve when I found out I was pregnant again. This time I still wasn't sure if everything would be okay. I then had to sit with an IV attached to my arm for three hours at the clinic because there was an experimental (unproven) treatment which would make it more likely for the baby to stick around. To be fair, if they'd said I had to eat Spam for every meal because it would help, I would have done it because after two miscarriages I was desperate for it to succeed. I didn't particularly enjoy being pregnant. I was paranoid when I couldn't feel the baby move. I would rush home from work and lie on my side in bed and drink cold water, waiting for the kicking to start. I went into hospital with cramps and was convinced I was having another miscarriage – I was embarrassed when I then had to inform my partner, the doctor and two nurses that the pain had gone because I'd done a massive poo and it must have been indigestion. I had expensive acupuncture where they burnt black stuff on my skin and asked me strange questions about my childhood. I went to a Tarot reader who told me the reason I couldn't have a baby was because I had issues with my dad and was set up for failure. She was wrong, obviously, as a) I did get pregnant and b) my dad was never a failure in my eyes. Let's just say, I don't feel like I had that kind of pregnancy where you walk about rubbing your tummy and smiling benignly like a lady in an advert for home insurance. I tried to be that woman and listened to lots of meditations and hypnobirthing soundtracks, but there was a voice that kept telling me that my pregnancy was too good to be true, I was too old to have a healthy baby and too greedy to want to have a baby at my age rather than just accepting that I'd had the career and the money and didn't deserve anymore, thank you.

When my daughter arrived, I felt like I'd survived the fertility challenge. I was in a great position to be a first-time mum. I was forty.

I was also broken and had nothing left to give.

NEWSFLASH: Being an older parent isn't easy

YES, I AM LUCKY, but that doesn't mean that I can't flag up some of the challenges of being an older mum. I will keep feeling lucky until I die, *but* new motherhood is hard.

So much of the focus when you're having fertility treatment is on getting pregnant. It's about the test, getting beyond twelve weeks, getting to twenty weeks, getting to full-term. There is no real focus on anything else, that is, the birth, bringing a baby home – bringing an actual baby home and looking after it – having a baby that turns into a child and bringing that child up, having a child that turns into a teenager and bringing that teenager up. It sounds naïve, but I remember standing in the supermarket in the baby aisle and looking up at all the different products – the formula milk, the weaning stuff, the nappies, the potties, training pants, school uniforms, exercise books, school bags – and just feeling utterly exhausted.

'But nobody told me that there was all this stuff too?' I said under my breath. There had been part of me that had only really envisaged a baby and perhaps I'd thought they just stayed as a baby, but of course what you have is a human that stays with you (if you're lucky) for the rest of your life and you are solely responsible for this human. It seems ridiculous that I hadn't realised this earlier, but I hadn't.

It's hard not to do the maths and think about how you'll be in a mobility vehicle by the time they start university. Not that there's anything wrong with mobility vehicles – it's just that you'll definitely be getting old at that point. One of the biggest challenges when you're older is the lack of stamina. The sheer gut-aching, bleary-eyed tiredness of motherhood.

When I was fifteen, I could readily drink a pint of Thunderbird (anyone who came of age in the late 80s will know what I'm talking about) and smoke twenty Silk Cut Extra Light and not feel terrible the next day. Fast forward to my forties and mid-forties and just looking at a glass of rosé gives me a hangover. Nobody had warned me that you don't sleep for about four years when you have children. I know I would have dealt with this lack of sleep much more easily if I'd been younger. Instead, it made me crazy, fly off the handle and question why on earth I'd made the decision to have children in the first place. Then I'd feel guilty because I was supposed to be LUCKY – and I was lucky, but I was also overwhelmed and tired and found it hard to cope.

Being an older parent is TOUGH. Don't be fooled by the celebrities who have kids in their late forties and early fifties – they have EXCELLENT CHILDCARE and are EYE-WATERINGLY RICH, and that takes the pressure off. These are the ways in which it can feel tough:

- You might not become a grandparent unless your kid decides to have kids young.
- You have to fight the instinct to lie down and only play games that involve lying down. My friend recommended 'day spa' as a good game as you can lie down and ask your kid to massage your face whilst you nap.
- Your moods can be unpredictable, especially if you have a baby but are also dealing with perimenopause.
- You've also had more life *without* kids than with, so the contrast of never having any ME TIME feels more extreme.
- You're also keenly aware that your time is limited on this Earth, so you're juggling children, work and all the other stuff (maybe trying to change careers, follow your dreams, move out of the rat race).
- Anything that can't be fitted in around nap times can be tough. For me that has meant hitting the breaks on writing and broadcasting because I've got a baby that has just woken up and doesn't like watching me work on a laptop.

'I have come to the realisation that I still have a lot of parenting to do and that's on top of everything else,' Clover Stroud said to me in an interview recently. She has five children and still manages to write books that are very good. There has been a lot written about the 'pram in the hall' (Cyril Connolly's famous quote about how having children is a barrier to 'good art'). One of the interesting things is that having limited time to write or do creative stuff can really focus your attention. At the moment I am writing this whilst one kid watches *Moon and Me* on TV and the other one dances around the kitchen to Ariana Grande. I have learnt to write in chaos and with lots of noise. I have had to fit writing in around small pockets of time (for me it often means putting one child on a screen and hoping the other one has a long nap).

I really try and ring-fence the small time I have and focus. I also think it's good for my children to see me prioritising the things I enjoy, like writing. All too often, mothers are martyrs and think they'll get an award for sacrificing all the things they love, when it only makes them miserable and resentful instead. In order to be able to give yourself over to being a parent, you need to feel like you have fulfilment in other areas of your life. I have spoken to mums who are desperately unhappy because they always put their own dreams and needs on the backburner and put off doing things 'until the children grow up'. Everyone has a different situation in terms of work, but I know that I have to spend some time doing the things I love or I can't focus on being a mum at all. Sometimes there are times when the two worlds are completely messy and blurred and that's when I tend to feel the most challenged – like I'm failing at my creative life, failing at work and being a crap mum at the same time. The main way I avoid this is putting my phone away when I'm with the kids (I try but often fail) and not looking at work stuff when I'm with them. It's a work in progress!

We need to talk more about infertility

A conspiracy of silence exists around becoming a mum later on in life, and the reality of fertility treatment and how it doesn't always work. Just as female celebrities don't talk about the fact they've had

Botox, they often don't talk about how they managed to have kids in later life. When I was trying to get pregnant the second time, I had a few people flag up that Janet Jackson had just had a baby aged fifty.

'See, you can get pregnant at any age,' someone would say; or, 'I had a friend who thought she was going through the menopause but actually she was pregnant and she was forty-eight!' When you're trying to get pregnant, there are hundreds of these stories that people tell you. They can drive you crazy but they are generally from well-intentioned people trying to cheer you up.

Celebrities aren't getting pregnant through ovulation kits or kale smoothies. Instead it's usually super-expensive fertility treatment or using a surrogate or adoption (requiring money, luck and lots of mental and physical resources). Although we don't need to OUT celebrity women about how exactly it happened, it's worth remembering that having kids in your mid- to late forties rarely happens naturally, and it's actually okay to not feel guilty about fessing up to it feeling difficult at times. We don't have to grin and bear it. We are lucky, but you can be lucky and exhausted at the same time.

The brochures focus on the happy, smiling faces of babies but they don't necessarily bring to life the challenging side of things. So, maybe it's worth us a) being realistic about what's involved so women can be readily prepared, and b) being honest about our route to parenthood so people don't think that it was easy and then feel bad because it's not easy for them.

I spoke to Cat Strawbridge who had ten rounds of fertility treatment and used to work at The Fertility Network, a support forum for women going through infertility. She has a podcast called 'Finally Pregnant' and also runs events for women in the midst of fertility treatment. Her journey to getting pregnant wasn't easy:

> I started trying to conceive in 2012 and nothing happened for a couple of years, during which time we went for some investigations.

Fast forward a long story and we ended up having three rounds of IUI [intrauterine insemination], four fresh rounds of IVF, two frozen transfers.

Just like many women she felt sure it would work right away:

I thought, 'I'm going to have a baby now' [after her first round], but IVF doesn't work 70 per cent of the time and often the first round can be investigative – trying to figure out what drugs work for you. If it doesn't work, it may be because some tweaks are needed. When I got pregnant, I thought we were sorted, but then we went for an early scan and realised there was no baby. The embryo had implanted, but there was no baby in the sac. That was awful. Going in and not thinking anything bad – just excited – that happening was awful.

Fertility treatment makes you feel invisible

There's a massive loss of identity for women going through IVF. Everything else fades into the background and you start to feel like the only thing that's going on is the struggle to get pregnant and the meetings at clinics and medical appointments.

'Relevance was a massive thing for me when I was going through it,' Cat says. 'I didn't feel relevant. I didn't know who I was. I wanted to create something where people felt relevant. We need reminding we have full lives so infertility doesn't take over everything.'

For me, I also had this feeling that I was underwater and everyone else was far away and I couldn't really hear what they were saying. My only focus was on whether the treatment would work or not. I became obsessive about getting pregnant and would often hide in the toilet and cry if another colleague announced they were pregnant. I just didn't feel like I was me anymore.

People give rubbish advice and everyone is a fertility expert

I was amazed at how tactless people were – saying things that I would never say to a woman trying to have a baby. Some friends would tell me how easy it was for them to get pregnant: 'I just have to take my pants off and I'm preggers.' Others would tell me to go on holiday and chill out (if I said we were trying). Others would tell me stupid, mythical stories about women who had got pregnant just when they were about to sign adoption papers or when they had a one-night stand with a younger man. THE WORST THING OF ALL WAS BEING TOLD TO RELAX. Having a needle shoved in your arm every morning to take blood is not relaxing. Having a *transvaginal ultrasound* shoved into your vagina three times a week is not relaxing (or at least it wasn't for me). Having to inject yourself with hormones in public toilets is not relaxing. Going to see an acupuncturist and being fleeced for £100. None of these things are relaxing.

Cat shared similar experiences:

> I once spoke to Dr Hilary, the TV doctor, and he told me to 'relax', and it seemed to perpetuate the useless advice offered. Relaxing is not going to get me pregnant. Sadly, there is so much useless advice. Someone might say that to someone who hasn't got fallopian tubes, [but] if you can't have babies medically, then how relaxed you are makes zero difference. When people tell you to 'go on holiday and it will happen', it's really frustrating. Also, when you've been trying, you never really stop trying. I [am] always quite aware of what's happening in my body and know when I'm ovulating. You can't forget about it.

Some women will obviously remain childless, but there isn't much chat about that either

There is support out there if you're going through this. The reality is that wanting kids and not having them is deeply traumatic. It's something that doesn't go away. I have had friends who've been through it and they're still processing what's happened. What they don't need is people telling them how much more carefree their lives are without kids, or people making patronising assumptions about how they get to lie in bed all day. A life without children is not easier – not if you wanted them, anyway. Cat feels it can be hard to meet other women in the same situation as it's potentially harder to spot:

> When you're a mum, you can see other mums and look at them across a room and know they are living a similar experience, but you can't see the people who haven't got children. There is no 'school gate', which can make it hard to find others who are in that situation too. I know people who have made peace with their childlessness. It doesn't leave though – the fact that you haven't had children. You grieve the scan pictures, birthdays, first day at school photos, then university, weddings, and then grandchildren. So, it goes on and on. If you want them but aren't able to have children, it affects your life profoundly.

Not having children when you dearly want them is one area that I haven't touched on so much in this book, but there is support and resources out there (you'll find these at the back of the book). The lessons, however, are clear. For some women, teaching them about bananas and condoms at school can seem pretty redundant when they find themselves twenty-five years later with their legs in stirrups being told 'There's nothing medically wrong with you but your eggs are probably a bit on the old side so you might not be able to have kids.' And let's be honest so that women know that fertility treatment presents many challenges – it's not easy and it won't always work, and there are other pathways to parenthood that we need to talk about so women can choose the best option. And finally, let's also share our experiences of being older mothers. Yes, we're lucky but it's hard and it's okay to say that and remember that adage 'WE CAN DO HARD THINGS' – it really helps on bad days.

CHAPTER FOUR

Why It's Okay to Listen to Radiohead, but Try and Dip Your Toe into New Music Too If You Can

This chapter is fairly short but it's important so don't skip it. Many of the reasons we feel old is because we stop doing the things we did when we were younger. One of these things is being open to new stuff. So that may be genres of film or books or music or it may be food or clothing or where you like to sit on a train (e.g. I have to be facing forwards, have a table and be 500 metres from the nearest toilet).

I realised quite recently that I was only listening to music from the 90s and noughties. I looked at Spotify and browsed the new artists and it was overwhelming. I was also worried about being a saddo and trying to reference Stormzy and people just thinking I was like the 'trendy' supply teacher we had at school (Mr Dudley) who used to ask us to call him Dave and wore novelty ties with Homer Simpson on. I was also worried that if I continued listening to the same music forever, I would get stale. And yes, it's fine to have preferences. Life is about making choices, trying things and discovering what you like, but there's a danger as we get into our forties and fifties that we get *too* set in our ways. I have noticed this with other older women. They complain that modern music is too sweary, then that the mustard on their burger isn't the right brand, that the napkin in the restaurant was crumpled, and the next thing you know they're supporting Brexit and think Nigel Farage is the Messiah. I'm kidding, but we sometimes put down the new stuff because it's intimidating and we like rolling around like an ageing pig in shit (though let's face it, Pulp were cool right? Or did you like Blur more?).

NB: Can I just say that I once attended a party in a hotel in East London and Jarvis Cocker was there. I had never been attracted to him before, but in the flesh (and I'd imbued some pharmaceuticals at the time) he was unnaturally attractive, so if he's reading this – and I'm guessing he might be as I'm imagining that he's been secretly following me on Instagram and is in love with me and has been for some time – then, Jarvis, PLEASE DO MESSAGE ME. My other half won't mind as I've said we should make exceptions for certain people (his is Kylie Minogue) and so we basically have this thing that is a 'celebrity open relationship' and we are free to sleep with celebrities if they proposition us (so far this hasn't been tested, which is a shame perhaps as we're both getting on a bit and could use some excitement).

Some quotes in my survey confirmed that a few of us feel like we're stuck in a rut:

> I feel like I rarely try anything new anymore.

> I'm not really sure where to start when it comes to new music and stuff.

There's a sense that our circle of influence gets smaller and smaller and we calcify. We can become rigid politically too – with strong beliefs that we've gleaned from only reading opinions that we agree with and only moving in circles with people who are just like us and mirror those opinions back in a pleasing manner (social media is like this).

Suddenly a few things started to happen to me music- and culture-wise. I'd always been an avid reader but I found when I looked at my shelves the books were all the same. There were lots of self-help books (and many were telling me *not to give a shit about anything* and to *not give a fuck* as this was a trend in books for a while). There were also books about women on a journey of self-discovery (i.e. Cheryl Strayed, Elizabeth Gilbert, Glennon Doyle). They were all good books but very 'samey' in their tone and message. Essentially, I was giving myself a continuous pep-talk and there wasn't much light and shade in there.

In my twenties and thirties, I'd cast my net wider and read lots of different authors. One of the reasons my behaviour changed is the fact that we live in a culture where we are constantly recommended things that we've previously liked before (i.e. Amazon telling you what your next book choice should be). This means we rarely experiment. It also means that if you're a white, middle-class woman, then you are possibly more likely to read books by white, middle-class women. Of course, these women get more opportunities (and I am privileged because I am one of them) because their books will be the ones that are recommended to you. You need to look beyond this or you will miss some very important things – politically, socially, culturally – and think that everyone is like you; and then you end up saying stupid stuff and not believing there are massive problems for people who are not like you, which there obviously are. I haven't elaborated on this here but if you're on social media, check how alike the people are that you follow and cast your net wider if you want to keep learning and growing, which is important.

Back in the eighties, friends gave me mix tapes. I would listen to albums all the way through and then go into record shops and try and browse all sorts of music – not just heading straight to the artists I already liked. I went to a lot of gigs (I can't remember the last time I went to see live music and Covid-19 obviously put a scupper on that as I'm writing this). I'd see a band a friend had recommended and sometimes they were awful and I'd never listen to them again, but there were a couple of occasions when I ended up loving these experiences. They opened my eyes.

As we age, we sometimes forget the passion that we once had for music. Or the way it feels to really immerse yourself in music (it may be that you only ever listen to music if you go running, rather than just seeing it as an activity in itself – something you can do in the evenings instead of watching TV, for instance). Our lives are busy and if we have kids then perhaps our days are overtaken with noise and we just long for silence. I recently realised that the only time I listen to music – like really listen versus just having the radio warbling away whilst I do chores – is when I go for a run. I kept wondering why I found my runs so transformative. Of course, there were the natural endorphins and the sensation of being outside, but it was also hearing music again, loud in my ears, and often music I'd loved in my twenties and thirties (with the odd track thrown in that I'd heard on 6Music and hurriedly searched for on Spotify). I now try and listen to music more at home and see it in the same way as having a bath or listening to a podcast. I can't say I've been out clubbing recently but I know that I want more of that feeling too (without the drugs) – more fun, more intensity, more forgetting my monkey-mind chatter and just abandoning myself to the moment. Once we're out of the woods – if we get out of the woods, Covid-wise – then I intend to go to a festival or a rave or even just a party, and dance rather than hover on the sidelines and then regret that I haven't at least tried to immerse myself in music the way I used to when I was younger.

Am I a cultural moron who is stuck in my ways and in need of shaking things up?

Here's a quick quiz… Are you ready?

- Do you feel like you lost ten years somewhere and still think All Saints were about ten years ago when their hit single 'Pure Shores' came out in 2000? And that's not ten years ago but TWENTY YEARS, right?

- Do you find it hard to listen to Radio 1 because all the songs seem really loud and make you feel anxious?
- Do you struggle to come up with five hits from the past twelve months?
- Do you find it hard to name someone under the age of forty who is a musician (and is not Ed Sheeran as he doesn't count)?
- Do you find yourself zoning out on a run when some old house music tune comes on and you're transported back to a chill-out room in Amsterdam and it's 1993 and you're watching a projector screen with a seagull flying in slow motion and someone is stroking your hair and saying that they love you over and over?
- Do you dance only if it's a fiftieth birthday and you've had two bottles of prosecco and someone plays Prince?
- Do you struggle to come up with your favourite film when someone asks and wonder whether it's okay to answer *E.T. the Extra Terrestrial*?
- Do you sometimes walk out of a shop because the music is too frenetic and you want something soothing and relaxing instead?

If you answered 'yes' to all of the above, then yes, you are just like me and in a cultural time warp

Your musical taste stalled somewhere in 2001 and you no longer have the capacity to absorb anything new or different. This can be incredibly ageing. It can make you sound like one of those music-bore men on BBC4 who talk endlessly about punk and how great it was and how there hasn't been any new musical phenomenon since then that came close. But the problem is, what's the alternative? Isn't it sad to try and stay up to date with what's hip now? (In fact, nobody actually says 'hip' do they?) Isn't it better to just stay in a bubble and listen to old Radiohead, Pulp and Prince and forget that anything has happened in the interim?

We need to fight getting stuck in our ways and keep trying new things

If we look at work, there are clearly things we decide about ourselves: we make assumptions about what we can't do and we often suffer from *imposter syndrome* (the idea that we aren't equipped to do the job and someone will discover we are stupid). We tell ourselves that we aren't good at certain things and then struggle to rid ourselves of that idea. For me the confidence issue was 'strategic thinking' – I thought I was hopeless at strategy despite the fact that I wrote dozens of presentations which demonstrated my strategic thinking. My mum always says that she hates games. 'There is nothing worse in the entire world than going to a party and having to play a game,' she proclaims. Now I have to agree that I'm not nuts about board games (I struggle to concentrate), but since having kids I've had to sit down and play UNO and Doggle. And what do you know? I quite enjoy them. It's relative: the kind of enjoyment you get from doing a wee in a service station toilet when you've been dying for the loo for ten minutes; not the kind of enjoyment you'd get from Brad Pitt snogging you.

The card game example might not be a good one as I realise it's not exactly the kind of hipster, exciting activity that feels like a challenge as we get older, but what I'm trying to say is IT'S IMPORTANT TO TRY NEW THINGS.

And don't make assumptions about what you can and can't do. Keep an open mind.

There are new things to try that will stop you feeling old

Your own list of things is going to be different dependent on what you currently do and like, but here are some suggestions:

Go into a shop with loud music and instead of running away, really listen

See if you can nod your head to the beat a bit. If you close your eyes, see whether you can access that feeling you used to get on a dancefloor back in the day. If a security guard looks at you weirdly, then just tell them you're going through the menopause and need a bit of space as you're feeling zoned out.

Spend a week listening to a different radio station

It doesn't matter what the genre of music is, as long as it's not what you've become accustomed to. I LOVE 6Music and listen to it religiously. I tell myself that this is keeping me youthful and abreast of new music (and it is because they do play a fairly mixed-up playlist), *but* I can now sing all the jingles and so I know I need to shake things up and try a different station (not necessarily a younger one, maybe just a different genre).

Eat things that you've always told yourself you hate

I have a partner who is quite set in his ways food-wise. Early on in our relationship he refused to eat a bacon sandwich because I'd put pepper in it (he chucked it in the bin and I cried because I'd made it for him and was overly sensitive in the first few months of our relationship). I've found that the older I've got, the more experimental I've become with food. There are two voices that are usually competing inside. Let's say we're sitting in a restaurant (these are different voices to the ones I talked about in the Botox story though – probably with different accents and maybe male instead of female).

> **Voice one:** *I will order the thing I always order because I know I like it.*
> **Voice two:** *Boring.*
> **Voice one:** *But what if I get the thing and I don't like it. I know that the thing I always get is the thing I like.*
> **Voice two:** *Jesus Christ.*
> **Voice one:** *Remember that time I tried that new thing and I was so disappointed and really wished I'd gone for my original order?*
> **Voice two:** *How old are you? 103? Go on then, old woman. Go with what you know.*
> **Voice one:** *Shut up. Okay. I'm going to order this thing that I've never tried. Even if I don't like it, it's a new experience and so I'm challenging myself in a minute, tiny way and so I can be proud of myself.*
> **Voice two:** *Whatever. You're sad. Bye.*

The trying new things off the menu analogy can actually be used in any situation. So, think about sex (if you actually have sex, which I don't – but that's a whole other book that I've co-written already, and I will have sex again eventually one day, I hope). Okay, you might think that going on top is not a thing that you do when you get older because your boobs hang down and your stomach looks like a crumpled carrier bag and your triple chin flops about as you look lovingly at your partner, who returns your gaze in horror, BUT how about giving it a try? (I haven't done this and am writing it as a dare for myself as I keep seeing women on top in Netflix series and wondering when was the last time I did this and realising it was twenty years ago at least.)

Watch a film that isn't recommended by your friends

When *Cats* came out, everyone panned it, and then one of my friends suggested going. I thought about the reviews, and yes it was actually pretty shit (and my friend thought so too, sort of), but I learnt something about myself: I don't like cats singing or feeling sexual attraction to cats singing because it makes me feel uneasy (as the owner of two cats who are very precious to me).

Don't get rigid in your thinking, and keep learning

This is a biggie. In this day and age it's very easy (because we all live in echo chambers) to only like people who agree with us and have a set of opinions that we've not really interrogated but have just come about through watching bits of TV shows or hearing someone we respect suggest something.

I have never been very interested in politics. This is not something I am proud of. In fact, I'm deeply ashamed. I grew up in the 1980s and hated Margaret Thatcher as much as the next kid, but my parents were very politically engaged and I rebelled and became an empty-headed imbecile who likes buying nice clothes. I am aware that I need to learn more about politics. I am also aware that I need to be very careful about how I'm forming opinions about stuff and where I'm getting my information from. My objective for the next few months is to learn more and talk less. Just as with every other area of our life, learning is a thing that we sometimes stop doing as we age. We just start accepting that things are true and not questioning them. And again, rigid is bad – nothing is ever set in stone. Okay, yes there are some concepts that are, but ideas and theories are always changing and evolving so it's important to keep learning and never feel like you've arrived already.

Taking a course is something to consider doing. There is a proliferation of online courses and they've made learning much more accessible. Learning doesn't necessarily need to mean signing up for a course, though. It also means buying a more challenging book which teaches you stuff on a topic that you've perhaps dismissed because you think it's not something you'll ever properly understand. I've spent much of my life telling myself that I'm no good at tech, no good at science, no good at maths, and I've avoided culture and literature in these areas. The truth is that this isn't actually true, or not entirely true, as I find a lot of science fascinating if it's told in a way that I can readily access and that isn't overly academic.

It's also important to follow people on social media who don't look like you and sound like you and live in the same situation as you. Listen and don't be quick to proffer an opinion. Think about stuff rather than getting yourself off the hook because you can't be arsed. This expands your horizons and hopefully will encourage you to take action, lend support and help to bring about change where you see injustices and challenges. This might be through sharing content or through actively demonstrating or through other means.

These are all things I am aware I need to do more of, and learning is part and parcel of the journey.

There are occasions when a rave track (recently it was Human Resource's 'Dominator') will come on the radio, and I will immediately be transported back to a sweaty club with lots of people grinding their teeth up and down (when clubs didn't smell awful because everyone smoked and it masked the smell of sweat) and me trying to find my boyfriend who's walked off (because he always used to walk off the minute we arrived anywhere and I'd spend the entire evening pretending this didn't bother me when really it did).

If 'Let The Beat Hit 'Em' by Lisa Lisa & Cult Jam comes on in the car, I'll stop thinking about sourdough bread toast and remember the night I got my eyelash extensions stuck in a wind machine and a beautiful transgender dancer had to help me, but then her wig got stuck and we ended up with a bouncer trying to help retrieve our self-esteem which had disappeared somewhere under the stage we were dancing on.

If I listen to The Orb and 'Little Fluffy Clouds', then I'm in a chill-out room at The Melkweg in Amsterdam and I'm watching a projector as it plays a strange bit of footage of a rabbit sitting on a car window screen who keeps jumping off and jumping back on again.

I remember sitting for over an hour watching this film and thinking I was learning something very profound. I heard 'Voodoo Ray' by A Guy Called Gerald when I was too young to go out properly but had dropped by a friend's house. Her big sister was talking about how they'd taken acid two nights previously and she'd been under the impression she could fly and had almost jumped off the balcony. The song made me feel nervous. It didn't sound like Brother Beyond or any of the other crappy pop bands I'd been listening to. (I thought INXS were experimental and hardcore because I'd got their album as a birthday present and played it so loud that my ghetto blaster speakers blew up.)

I remember hearing 'Cascades' by Sheer Taft at my friend Diana's house (she sadly died soon afterwards of a brain aneurysm). We were getting ready to go out and jumping around with butterflies in our tummies and I was trying to wrestle my feet into some size 5 white platform sandals that I'd bought in Waterlooplein market earlier that day with the proceeds from my cleaning job.

I sometimes imagine myself in an old people's home in the future with Orbital coming on the radio (it won't be a radio – it will be a virtual screen with holographs or avatars or whatever shit is actually happening), and all us old, ex-party people standing up, wobbly at first, some clutching our walking frames, and slowly moving to the middle of the carpeted dining room and raising our arms in the air and swirling around and punching the air, and the care-workers telling us to go and sit back down and making a mental note never to play Orbital again. This idea makes me smile. It also makes me want to go and watch Orbital – not as a forty-seven-year-old but as I was back in the summer of whatever the hell it was when I was wearing a turquoise mini-dress that my friend Martje made me, with a matching glittery rucksack and those white platforms.

Things I miss about my youth

- Being able to get out of bed without something hurting.
- Feeling like any minute my life will change for the better but not realising I have any role to play in this myself.

- Smoking.
- Snogging.
- A lot of time staring at the ceiling pondering (no smart phone back then).
- Getting a pizza slice for a pound at Piccadilly Circus and eating it whilst waiting for the night bus (I don't miss the night bus but I do miss the pizza late at night).
- Being sick in clubs but then getting back on the dance floor as if nothing had happened.
- Thinking I might live in Hollywood one day (but taking no steps to actually make this happen).
- No hangovers.
- Not having to wear a bra.
- Actually looking okay.
- Having a waist.
- Going to see bands and heading right to the front, then trying to get eye contact with the lead singer and 'fainting' so I can perhaps get backstage. I did this at the 'Capital Radio Junior Best Disco' when Johnny Hates Jazz came on (not that I liked them – I'd heard Curiosity Killed The Cat were in the VIP area, but they weren't and I ended up in a St John's Ambulance wrapped in one of those silver blankets and unable to get back inside the venue).
- Talking for hours on the landline.
- Talkabout (if you know, you know).
- Listening to a whole album and rewinding it and listening to it again.
- Listening to the Top 40 on Sunday and being genuinely excited to find out what might be Number 1.
- Holding hands with a boy.
- Going out with £10 to spend for a night out and coming home with £2.
- The Body Shop pineapple face wash.

Why we need to embrace our ANGER

When I was a child, I often got very angry about small things (like most kids do). Dad used to tell a story of taking me into a toy shop in Hamilton, Ontario, where we lived. I was probably about three years old and I wanted this specific teddy bear and he wouldn't buy it so I flung myself on the floor. Then, as he tried to drag me out the door (there was none of the apologetic/ placating parenting that we all tend to fall victim to nowadays), I sank my tiny milk teeth into the wooden door frame. Dad was scared that if he pulled too hard my teeth would come out in the door frame so he instead tried to talk me out of biting a hole in the door (so furious was I). Eventually he managed and my teeth were intact and I lived to bite again. In primary school I bit a girl who refused to share her Lego with me. I still remember the look of shock and pain in her face as I sank my teeth into her chubby arm. Mrs Green then asked me why I did it and I shrugged my shoulders. Shrugging shoulders was seen as incredibly rude if you were a kid in the 80s and so I was made to stand in the corner of the class with my hands on my head until it was time for my grandad to come and collect me. This was for about three hours, which is barbaric if you really think about it, but I stopped biting people so I guess it worked.

I'm not advocating that women turn to biting when they get angry, but it's strange that over the years I've learnt how to contain my anger, how to turn it inwards, how to turn it on myself so I say hateful things to myself, how I've shoved it away so it doesn't harm others. I was taught by society that being an angry woman was unattractive. Angry women were to be ridiculed. I remember seeing TV sitcoms where angry women would drag their husbands out of pubs and the men would roll their eyes because there was simply nothing more silly than a woman shouting and screaming her head off. Or angry women were put into asylums. Women were supposed to be agreeable and shouldn't lose their tempers. All through my twenties and thirties I'd absorbed these messages and so I became a doormat with a 'Walk all over me please' sign scrawled on my forehead. The anger was still there. I got angry when a guy I'd been snogging shoved his hand in my pants without warning and tried to push me into a car park to have sex with me (I managed to run away). I got angry when colleagues took credit for work I'd done. I got angry when I failed to get pay rises and saw male colleagues doing less work getting them. I got angry when I had to go through fertility treatment. I got angry when I felt I was discriminated against because I was a mum and my senior role at work no longer existed. I shoved that anger inside. It turned to anxiety and low-level depression and a feeling I had that my life wasn't how it should be but I couldn't do anything about it.

When I look back on those years, I realise that the women I admired were often angry ones. I had a massive crush on Courtney Love and listened to Hole incessantly. I liked Skin from Skunk Anansie. I also loved Brody Dalle from The Distillers (but was jealous because she was married to Josh Homme). Sometimes during long work meetings with men launching into one-hour monologues about the *semiotics of disposable dish cloths* I'd ask myself, 'What would Courtney Love do?' (I still think this is a good title for a self-help book – I'd buy it). Courtney would be in that meeting and she'd get up, wearing a ripped-up nightie and her guitar over one shoulder, she'd upturn the board room table, then she'd shove that boring man against the glass window and she'd scream in his face, 'SHUT UP, YOU FUCKING BORING WANKER! YOU ARE TALKING BOLLOCKS AND I CAN'T LISTEN TO ONE MORE WORD OF THIS SHIT!' Then she'd perhaps take a swig from a bottle of Jack Daniels and shove two fingers up at everyone and swagger out again – ready to perform at Earls Court. She would not apologise. She would not turn her anger inside and let it chew her all up.

I was in awe of women like her. I wanted to be like them. It gave me headaches – the repressed anger that I'd kept inside for so long. It wasn't healthy. The thing is, anger is often a symptom that something is wrong and if you keep pushing it away, you're essentially never going to work out what that thing is. Anger can often be positive in showing you a way forward. There are obviously different types and now that I'm in my forties I can distinguish between them. Low-level anger that is usually provoked by something quite petty, like a friend not inviting me to a social and then telling me a fib. Then there is hormonal anger, which is before my period and is set off by anything (e.g. a half-digested carrot that hasn't been picked up or a row of cat biscuits wedged between the floorboards). There's also sleep deprivation anger, which is frightening in its intensity and can only be unleashed by acts of violence. As I don't want to hit my children, I tend to break things, toss things in the bin that are getting on my nerves or throw things out the window (usually my partner's socks or the hat he uses after he washes his hair to keep his hair flat).

Let's just say that I've come to accept my anger and I try harder to interrogate it and ask questions like 'Why am I angry?', 'What can I do with this anger?', 'What will make it better?', 'What action can I take?' And I refuse to shove it inside and swallow it up, because I know that is too damaging. I still find myself getting overwhelmed at times but there are some tangible ways that you can calm down if you find yourself flinging stuff about the place:

- **Breathing:** I did a bit of research on this and discovered that when we get angry we tend to breathe more rapidly. This sets off our *fight or flight response* and the body is flooded with adrenalin and cortisol, which is what we need if we're about to run away from a bear but is not what we need if we're trying to find a school cardigan and have two minutes until school drop-off. The first step is to focus on the breath. There are apps that can help with this but one of my favourite techniques is 'alternate nostril breathing', which I learnt from an online yoga video. I won't explain it in detail here, but look it up and give it a whirl. My family know I'm battling anger if I'm hiding in the toilet doing this.

- **Notice what the voice inside is saying to you:** When I'm angry, the voice inside – the inner critic, whatever you want to call it – is shouting abuse. It's saying things like 'THIS HOUSE IS A FUCKING TIP! NOBODY CARES! I CAN'T STAND THIS PLACE! THIS ENTIRE FAMILY SUCKS!' It's also shouting insults at me, saying things like 'THIS IS YOUR FAULT. YOU CREATED THIS. AND NOW YOU'VE SHOUTED AT EVERYONE AND YOU'RE A USELESS PARENT.' When you listen to this voice, like really listen, then you realise how absurd it is. Sit down. Interrupt the voice and say, 'THANK YOU FOR YOUR INPUT, BUT CAN YOU FUCK OFF QUIETLY SO I CAN CALM THE FUCK DOWN?' I also do this with anxiety and any other emotion that gets that inner voice worked up.
- **Do some exercise:** This helps because after exercise your body is full of endorphins and is less likely to be triggered by mess (for me it is often mess that sends me into a full-blown rage).
- **Think about what triggers your anger:** Once you've calmed down, see if you can identify a pattern in terms of what sets you off. So, yes, mess is one of my triggers. Then there's the weekday mornings when I need to get out of the house quickly and nobody's listening to my pleas to get dressed/brush teeth/etc. The other triggers are my partner not looking at me when I'm talking to him, WhatsApp (especially those messages that relate to school updates), cats that try and sit on me when I've just sat down and need

space, rude people on public transport, rude bosses who bark orders and have expectations that are way too high, etc. Once you know what triggers you, you'll feel more in control because you can try breathing and being mindful in these particular situations and give yourself a pep talk: 'Yes, this is a trigger, yes you usually get angry, but let's try breathing and stopping that inner critic and see if we can break the pattern today, okay?'

- **Channel the anger into something:** This could be writing. A good practice when you feel out of control is actually grabbing a pen and writing everything down that you're feeling in the moment and venting. The only thing to watch out for is that other people might read this if you leave it lying around. My mum once found an old diary and inside I'd written that I wanted to throw her down the stairs. This wasn't very nice and I had to explain that I'd written it aged 15 and had just found I'd been grounded and couldn't go to a 'Brother Beyond' concert in Islington. You can also channel anger into other things like painting or playing an instrument or even tidying up.

- **Try listening to something:** This could be music, or a meditation app, or anything that makes you appreciate the moment and calms you down.

We need to make friends with our anger. We need to sit it down and bite it on the arm. We need to accept it. We need to ask it what it needs us to do and not ignore it. We need to interrogate it and question why as women we are made to feel so bad about getting angry. It's actually a normal emotion just like sadness, worry, excitement, etc.

NB: If you have serious anger issues, then seek professional help (i.e. your GP or a therapist). Don't bite people.

CHAPTER FIVE

How to Master Your Work Demons and Learn from Millennials (Rather than Bitch about Them and Feel Jealous)

Women often feel invisible in the workplace as they get older – they lose their confidence and often lack self-esteem. There is a lot of ageism and discrimination, and women who have been away from work (having kids or taking a career break) can feel utterly irrelevant when they return.

Some quotes from my survey brought this to life:

I think women are discriminated in the workplace at either end of their career. There seems to be a sweet spot in your late twenties and then you hit your stride in your thirties, but it often gets interrupted by pregnancy, and when you want to get back to it, you're too old. It's rubbish!

I thought I'd feel more confident when I was older, but the truth is everyone is now younger than me and they don't have kids and can work differently to me. Also, it feels like a lot of my skills have gone out of fashion!

I found being at work really demoralising. Everyone seemed more clever, and I noticed people just ignored me or put me in the 'mum club' so didn't give me interesting stuff to do.

How we need to adapt and learn in order to master the new world of work

I worked in the same job for seventeen years. This in itself is a weird anomaly and I realise I sound like a dinosaur in today's climate of side hustles and freelancing and changing roles every couple of years.

The world of work that I entered was very different to the one we find ourselves in now (and to be frank, as I'm writing this in the midst of Covid-19, it's already the case that there's greater job insecurity).

The old world of work

Technology was entirely different when I started work in the late 90s. We had paper diaries that we wrote our appointments in (giant leather ones and of course there were Filofaxes – I always wanted one of those but never could afford one). Mobile phones were a novelty and people laughed if they saw someone talking in the street on one. There was email and faxing, but the pace of work was far slower. It wasn't unusual to send an email and not hear back for a day or two. It wasn't quite like carrier pigeon but there definitely wasn't the idea that you had to reply the minute you saw something in your inbox. So, you didn't start grinding your teeth and pacing up and down if you didn't get a reply. You didn't hit refresh over and over just to double check if you'd somehow missed this reply. You didn't take your phone with you to the canteen so you could hunch over it to press refresh over and over, wondering 'WHY ON EARTH HAS THIS PERSON NOT RESPONDED ALREADY?' The stress was there. There were still difficult clients and a clear hierarchy (clearer than today when it's sometimes hard to determine who the boss is because nobody wears shoulder pads anymore or has their own office). In the market research world in which I worked, there was a clear chain of command. When you started, you were basically somebody's BITCH and you carried stuff and made tea and agreed to everything they said and didn't speak unless you were spoken to. You were in charge of the projector, making sure everything was printed up and pouring water if people were thirsty. You moved up the ranks slowly (maybe progressing to the next level in 2–3 years) but not until you'd got all the bits of your job description ticked off.

As a young woman looking up at boss level, I struggled to find role models. The men seemed to be under the impression that they were Hollywood film directors, when in fact they were working on dog food strategy in Poland. Some of the senior women had had their empathy skills forcibly removed so they could be more competitive (perhaps because they had to do this – it was hard because female bosses were usually seen as horrible bitches and played to type). As I became more senior, I found meetings impossible to navigate. Was I supposed to whack my fist on the table and chat about golf? Or should I say nothing and then quote some French philosopher like some of my male colleagues did and which seemed to work in their favour? (NB: I had one male colleague who always managed to throw a reference to Baudelaire into client meetings. It made him come across as intellectually superior. Twat.)

The old world of work was dominated by masculine codes and the women that did well were the ones who learnt how to adapt. Or they knew their place (mine was pouring tea/water and being a sympathetic ear).

The new world of work

Fast forward to today, and the world of work couldn't be more different. We work longer hours and there isn't a sharp division between home and work. Technology allows us to work anywhere but that also means it's impossible to switch off. If you don't reply to an email within a certain time frame, then people assume you are a slacker. There is not so much time to think about stuff, and the focus is on churning out emails and going through endless tick lists that seem to get longer each day. The timelines of projects are quicker. I've struggled as an older woman with small kids. I've worked in agencies and I've freelanced. The freelancing is impossible with small kids as childcare isn't flexible enough to be able to just book in a couple of hours here or there. In agencies I felt out of place because everyone was so wedded to their work and more technically savvy than I was. I also got exasperated by the expectation that one should be present in the office and the sense that I had to sit there until 5pm even if my work for the day was done (and I'd skipped lunch so I could get out of work early).

Covid-19 has interestingly changed some of this rigidity because employers have been forced to let people work from home. So, there is reason for optimism and it's not yet clear where we will net out – whether things will go back to how they were or they will change. I spoke to Annie Auerbach, author of *FLEX: Reinventing Work for a Smarter, Happier Life,* and founder of Starling trends agency, about the impact it might have on working practices. This is what she said:

> One thing that has come out of this incredibly anxious, fraught pandemic period, is that remote working has gone from being a privilege for the few, to tipping over into the mainstream. The businesses that insisted flexibility wouldn't work have had to rush to adapt new flex ways of working, so I hope that there will be an easier path to flex from now on. Rigid set hours, long commutes and all being in the same place at the same time for five days a week seems absurd when we have proved again and again that people thrive when they have autonomy over their own time and are trusted to work in ways that work for them. Productivity goes up, wellbeing increases, staff retention goes up.

It remains to be seen whether any of these changes will stay in place, but arguably more flexibility around where we work is a good thing and something that was nigh-on unheard of when I was entering the work force. Interestingly, I recently had a role that in theory felt more flexible because it was working from home, but I found that the level of work required was entirely unmanageable. Online tools were used to micro-manage every moment of time, and as soon as the day's tasks were completed, new tasks popped up in their place. The language used by the staff was mechanical – it was about 'having capacity' and 'task completion'. It almost felt as if there was a robot manager taking over my life. This worried me as it made me think that technology and the ability to monitor output and productivity were being used to create unhealthy work practices. Sometimes it still feels as if technology is offering us flexibility, but if it isn't managed in an empathetic way, it threatens to push work into every area of our life.

Millennials versus Generation X

One of my roles in my old job was to look after people – manage their careers and their objectives and ensure they got the kind of exposure they needed to thrive. There was this constant tension between the Millennials and Gen X and Millennials were more demanding and impatient to move up the ladder. They were seen as being hard to manage because they didn't respect the old rules of work. They didn't KNOW THEIR PLACE. This was particularly true for the women who asked for promotions, pay rises and didn't sit quietly in meetings massaging the male egos or pouring the tea. There was less of a hierarchy, so my younger work colleagues weren't happy to take notes or schlep heavy bags or go and get coffee. This was a big bugbear for managers – they'd spent their entire careers doing grunt work (the women anyway) and couldn't understand why these spring chickens wouldn't SUCK IT UP. There was a sense of imbalance, so younger women were far more adept at technology and understanding intuitively how to get stuff done quickly and efficiently *but* they didn't always have the people skills to get along with teams/managers/clients. Interestingly, this is the stuff – the people stuff – that can take time to wrap your head around.

When I returned from my first maternity leave, I was BLOWN AWAY by how confident the younger women in my team were:

They asked for more money.
They said if they weren't happy.
They asked for promotions.

And I'll be honest and say that it inspired feelings of jealousy (and awe).

My own career progression had been slow and tedious, and I'd spent a lot of time doing stuff that really wasn't enjoyable. For example, taking packets of biscuits out of their packaging and then ironing the packaging so it could be mounted onto cardboard (doing this exercise for ten different countries meant in total I had to iron about a thousand pieces of biscuit packaging). In the beginning my envy of the younger women didn't serve me well. I got grumpy. I picked faults. I was too uptight to open up and say what was bugging me. I also felt on the backfoot technology-wise. As you will read in other chapters, the secret to not getting old and fuddy-duddy is to remain flexible and open to new ideas. I found it hard to do this. I still find it hard sometimes. I have to remind myself that just because my working life was different doesn't mean that the next generation will put up with it too. They have every right to shape their own destinies and demand more. But the question remains: WHO WILL ACTUALLY MAKE THE TEA? IS IT ME?

These are some of the things I told myself during this time:

I am hopeless at technology.
I don't deserve a pay rise or any recognition.
I don't know why someone would hire someone like me as I'm
older than everyone else and am out of the game.

And this is how I looked at younger female colleagues:

Who does she think she is? She's referencing social media accounts I've
never heard of and some platform that hasn't even been invented!
Look at her SKIN! When did my skin stop glowing?
Does she expect ME to take all the notes? When I started off, I
had to spend hours writing notes during meetings and then typing
them all up and circulating them, yet she does nothing but just says
something clever about 'BIG DATA' and she's suddenly a genius.

I often spoke to these women and knew they had the same imposter syndrome and insecurities as me. They were just better at disguising their feelings and forging ahead. They'd been told they could achieve anything and didn't let the fact that they were entering uncharted territory paralyse them.

THEY WERE INSPIRING.

In contrast, I was often stuck. I had a lot of old narratives in my head (these are still in my head as I write this chapter) about the things I was less capable of doing, despite having a podcast, writing books, being hired for new jobs *and* heading up a massive company for two years. I had read all the profiles of 'confident' older women and yet there were, and still are, days when I feel I'm lousy at everything I do. Sometimes women (especially my generation of women who grew up in a relatively sexist work culture) need to be reminded that they are good enough and that their experience is valuable but at the same time, there's a need to keep abreast of new stuff and not stick to familiar territories. The new world of work feels overwhelming at the best of times, but if you're also navigating being a parent, going through the menopause, feeling like your face is sliding off... Well, it just makes coping with new stuff quite challenging.

The problem is that sometimes younger people *are* better – not in all ways but in some. They are better for two reasons: first, they have more enthusiasm and are less jaded; second, they are more agile and keen to learn new stuff and embrace new challenges rather than telling themselves they won't be able to do it. And, yes, there will always be younger people who are more appealing to an employer because they're cheaper to hire and usually don't have children yet (having children is still viewed as a negative by the vast majority of employers).

One of the things I've noticed about people who age well and seem energised and interesting is their ability to adapt to new circumstances. The opposite of this is those who are rigid and have very defined ideas about what they like and don't like/what they can and cannot do. I talked about this in Chapter Four. It's good for you to keep evolving and not listen ONLY to Radiohead, even if they were/are a great band. I've felt myself swinging in this direction at times, especially when it comes to work – for example, telling myself that I'm no good with technology, when I haven't always made an effort (in actual fact, I am not too bad at it). I also have a lot of negative thinking tied up with my old job and the things I was told there – for example, I always thought I wasn't bright enough because I didn't go to Oxford or Cambridge (I was the only non-Oxbridge employee when I was hired) and I wanted so badly to be liked that I avoided ever saying anything remotely controversial.

Work and anxiety

For much of my career I accepted that feeling on edge and anxious was the norm. I got butterflies in meetings. Hid in toilets with my head in my hands. Cried on my way home. At that time, people didn't talk about mental health, and the predominant business model was that you put your 'game face' on and basically pretended everything was okay. There were days when my anxiety wasn't ramped up 100 per cent, but I now realise that I was feeling very uncomfortable for much of the time and couldn't put my finger on why. The thing is, the masculine (rigid) culture of work, the fact that so much priority was placed on being strong, domineering and loud, just wasn't in tune with my personality. I can be loud but I need to feel like I'm in a safe environment and not one where I'll get criticised the minute I express an idea.

This anxiety doesn't go away in our forties; in fact, it can often ramp up, the reason being that as well as the usual work pressures, such as working with difficult people and speedier timelines for projects, we question whether we're good enough and whether our opinions matter, because we're feeling less relevant and capable than others. I've learnt that the kind of team you have and the people who manage you are super-important. If you have someone who acknowledges that you feel on the back foot at times, someone with empathy, you can really flourish. However, if you have a manager that only points out what you can't do rather than praising what you can… Well, those old feelings of unworthiness and imposter syndrome return.

I have gone in and out of agency roles and recently went back into one which reminded me of how important a supportive and empathetic team can be. I quickly lost confidence in my ability and started to create my own negative narratives. I dreaded Monday mornings. I had a boss who used technology to manage every minute of my time. There was a perception that each day should be filled with tasks and once they were done there was 'capacity' to take on more, like a machine rather than a person. I was only told what I was doing wrong (and these things were minor details). I dreaded each catch-up. The problem was exacerbated by the fact that we only worked remotely and so the sole steer I had were the endless comments on my work. This meant that documents were often revised multiple times, which never gave the reward or dopamine rush of having finished something or a *job well done*. It didn't help that both my kids were at home for some of this working time and I was barricaded in a bedroom upstairs, listening to them screaming whilst just about to hop on another 'feedback Zoom'. I had to get out.

One thing that happens when you're older is that you're less willing to compromise everything for a job and are better able to recognise when it's not working out. It was risky for me to quit as I had no new job lined up, but I knew my mental health was getting worse, I was starting to question the things I did outside of work, like my podcast and my writing. I knew if I stayed, I'd be in a serious professional slump that would take some time to dig myself out of.

However, there are times when you can't leave for financial reasons. This sense of being 'stuck' in a job and feeling high levels of anxiety is really stressful. It is easy to feel overwhelmed and like things are never going to get any easier, but there are still things you can do.

It's okay to ask for help

Another thing that can increase anxiety at work is when you feel like you're out of your depth because your skills are a little dusty. Sometimes I'll avoid doing certain tasks because I'm worried I'll fail. This becomes problematic because people think you're flaky and lazy when actually you're scared. This can be difficult if you're in a senior role and the expectation is that you know everything.

One thing I've tried to do is ask a colleague for help – someone who has the skill that I lack. A recent example was a complex, Excel document (I have told myself for many years that Excel is not my friend). Each time I tried to type into it, the boxes would come out of alignment and I was wasting hours trying to get it to look okay. I started to feel desperate and the voice inside was saying, 'You're crap at Excel. You can't do anything technical. You're wasting too much time on something that should be straightforward, etc.' I asked my colleague if they could offer me some hacks so I could get a bit speedier, and then my colleague needed help writing and editing a blog that was due up that day for the social media feed. It was a win/win as both of us learnt new skills and next time I know I won't be so scared of working on Excel and can start to change some of those negative narratives in my head.

A lot of female friends kick off their conversations about work by telling me all about the stuff they can't do well. This is a typical female trait, whereas men are more likely to focus on the stuff they can do (or maybe they just give that impression to the outside world and inside they're quaking in their boots?). If it's something that you want to get the hang of and you feel continually on the back foot, then talk to your employer. You should not be penalised for needing to refresh some of your skills, especially if you've been away from the workplace on maternity leave or are new to a role. Remember the key to not getting too stuck in your ways is to keep learning, keep moving forward and remember you still have the capacity to adapt and try new things.

Positive self-talk

There can be a tendency, when you lose confidence, to start telling yourself a lot of negative shit. That awful voice starts up, the one that sounds like your mum/teacher/bully at school. You analyse your past and think about the times you've failed and the mistakes you've made, and you label the movie that's playing 'I Have Always Sucked at Work'. The truth is you have many talents. Performance is rooted in the way you feel about yourself. If you have a Zoom presentation, and just beforehand you tell yourself that you're going to mess it up, that your chin looks flabby, that your charts aren't good enough, that nobody on the team likes you, then the likelihood is that things won't go your way. If I have a big presentation (and a lot of my job revolves around presentations), I sometimes stand for a moment with my hands on my hips and say, 'You've got this!' I actually have a lovely sign where I work (in my bedroom) that a friend sent me that has this message embroidered on it. If the negative chatter persists, if I've received some mixed feedback, if a meeting hasn't gone as well as planned, I use whatever tools that I have available to perk myself up again. This might be a hot bath (if working from home – you can do this instead of taking a lunch break, and it really works) or a walk outside (to regain perspective) or a short meditation.

Sometimes this negative chat can also extend to constantly moaning about your job to anyone you meet. I've been in this situation several times and have talked to complete strangers in the park about how awful my boss is, how unmanageable my workload is and how depressed I am. This moaning doesn't help. Or it might help initially, but you'll find that ultimately it makes you feel drained (and others too). Instead, try and get out of the fixed mindset of 'This is intolerable' and move to a growth mindset and think 'How can I make this more tolerable?' or 'How can I plan my next move towards something better?' Do a bit of moaning and then take action.

Try a life/career coach

Sometimes when you're stuck in a job that you hate, it can feel like you're paralysed and there's no end in sight. The idea that you might be able to find a new direction or 'pivot' appeals, but it's impossible to see the steps you need to take to get out of one role and into another. Social media can compound the sense that everyone's professional lives are going swimmingly, whilst you're in the minority, floundering in the '*hate my job*' shallows. In the past I've used a life coach to help me clarify what I want. This helped in several ways: first off, it made me feel like I was doing something positive in terms of changing my life IN THE MOMENT and wasn't just wallowing with no hope of anything getting better; it also helped me break down in manageable steps how I could move to a happier professional life.

I found a life coach was helpful because she held me accountable and each week asked me whether I'd done the things we'd agreed on during the previous call. She set me objectives. These things were often tied up with understanding my finances and how I spend money on luxury corduroy dungarees, which means I'm in more debt and have to do jobs I hate. She taught me that I was spending beyond my means and moving further away from the life I wanted. I am currently freelancing and trying to balance that with writing and developing my business. I have not achieved a perfect balance but I am on my way and feel more of a sense of agency over my professional life. Before, I had this idea that someone would swoop down (preferably someone who looked like the late Michael Hutchence) and carry me off on a chariot so I could sit in their palace, with my flashy new laptop, eating Ferrero chocolates and writing bestsellers all day. (If you are this person, then I'm still open to this idea, especially if you have a heated pool and live in a hot climate.)

Life coaches often offer free sessions if they're still training, or there are taster sessions that are free. I go on personal recommendation, so it's worth asking friends if they know of anyone; alternatively, look on social media at people who are recommended and see if their approach is what you're looking for. I've found that some can be a little vague/airy-fairy, so you need to find one that has the right philosophy for you and can tell you what difference they'll make to your professional life.

Don't let the bastards get you down

I have a small card that my dad gave me with this message on the front. In any job there are likely to be difficult personalities. People who suck at empathy. People who have unrealistic expectations in terms of deadlines. People who fail to notice that you wrote an entire report in two hours and point out that the page numbers should be centred rather than to the right. I have worked with a myriad of difficult personalities and at times have let these people dominate my life. I've dreaded going into work or joining a call because I know this person will be there.

There is no hard and fast solution to working with these people, but one thing you need to try and do is separate the fact from the fiction. If they're critical of you, is anything they say grounded in fact? If it is, then how can you work on those skills and perform better next time? Is there some training you can ask for or an expert in that area that you can quiz? If there is no evidence to support their critical point of view, then talk to a colleague you trust and see if they have had similar experiences. Nine times out of ten you'll discover that this person is difficult and the criticism isn't a true reflection of your performance. One of the benefits of ageing is that I am now more confident in calling people out if they treat me badly at work. In the past I would have internalised it all and cried and lost sleep. Now I am more likely to launch an investigation and talk to others (to see if they've also had negative experiences). If there is a particular example where I feel the person has treated me unfairly, I speak to them about it. I do take constructive feedback but I'm more likely to push back if I feel they're being critical for the sake of it. I'll also go and speak to Human Resources.

Be clear on what you can and can't do

It's simple. You need to say 'no' sometimes and be clear on what you can and can't do. I had a boss who micro-managed me and would also set a time limit in terms of when she expected things to be delivered. So, she'd say that I had two and a half hours to write a report and no longer than that. I was very clear when she told me this: yes, I could work on the report for two and a half hours and then I would send it to her in whatever state it was in (because the likelihood would be that it wouldn't be formatted, finalised and spell-checked). Alternatively, she could let me finish the report to the best standard – this might take a little longer but ultimately would require less work her end so would in fact save time.

Ultimately, if your current work situation isn't working, then start planning your escape strategy. If you can't get out at the moment, then look at the big picture and visualise where you want to be in five years' time. Try and take tiny, incremental steps to get there. Don't give up.

A note on redundancy: As I write many people are being made redundant or face the prospect of it happening soon because of the impact of the global pandemic. I have taken voluntary redundancy and been made redundant once. If you're already suffering from imposter syndrome and age-related work anxiety, it can be super tough. My advice is to use all the tools that you can to stay optimistic: keep to a routine, eat healthy food, meditate, get outside or do whatever keeps you on a steady-ish keel, keep applying for jobs, put as many feelers out there as you can and don't give up. There is no magic wand I can wave to make it better (I wish there was), but you will get back on top of things eventually. You *will* (I also send you a giant hug).

How older women can get with the new work vibe

Now there may be plenty of older women out there who think they've got everything sussed work-wise. These are the women who get up at 4.30am, do Pilates, drink smoothies, have an app that they've designed themselves in their spare time, and check emails whilst they're preparing dinner for their eight children.

If this is YOU, then you probably don't need to read this chapter. OR THIS BOOK.

Instead I'm talking to the women who feel like they've lost their confidence work-wise – like they don't feel like they're in the cut and thrust, that after having kids they struggle to stay motivated at work – and who sometimes look at younger colleagues in awe and can't figure out how they have all the success. The women who basically feel a big, fat LACK when it comes to work.

I am talking to you because this is me – most of the time – even now.

Even though I know I'm clever (but even as I write this my cheeks are burning with embarrassment) and can do cool things and have great ideas, I've found that as I've aged, my insecurities have grown. Recently I had to write a market research presentation – it was the kind of thing I've done hundreds of times. I have worked on and off in market research for eighteen years. The week leading up to the debrief, the negative voices started in my head. I started telling myself that I couldn't work the technology, couldn't access the platform to get the data, couldn't understand the data, couldn't deal with the new template which was unfamiliar, couldn't write clear and concise charts, couldn't present to the client over the phone and couldn't get approval from my senior colleague because she'd think my work was shit. This was the garbage I told myself and it was exhausting.

And it's strange because the survey I carried out revealed a similar pattern. Yes, many women said they felt more confident and cared less about what others thought (implying maybe less self-doubt and critique) but then there were also loads of comments like this:

I feel like a failure in about every aspect of my life.

I worry about job prospects and up-and-comers from the younger generation. They're so full of confidence!

I like the idea of feeling more confident, but it hasn't happened yet.

I would like to say that I'm confident but I just haven't got there yet workwise.

Sadly, many of us feel we're lacking when it comes to our job skills and think we can't 'compete' with younger colleagues. Sometimes this might be because we've been away from the workplace for a while, or it might be because we're still holding onto negative things we were told in the past. It is an internal narrative that we're all playing ourselves: *I'm not relevant. I'm out of touch. I don't know how to do this stuff.*

What can we do to turn this around?

Collaboration is a positive way forward

Instead of seeing younger women as competition, it's more constructive to think about what skills you have and what skills they have so you can collaborate together. I spoke to Emma Gannon, a writer and broadcaster who has written extensively about the new work culture and what it takes to succeed. She proffered up some good advice for older women at work.

> I have definitely been on the receiving end of that competitive energy in one of my first jobs with a female boss. In my book *The Multi-Hyphen Method* I talk a lot about how these generational divides are quite unnecessary – we have so much to learn from each other, and we have so much more in common than we think. I don't like to make generalisations but I do think it's down to an element of historic tension. In the era that my boss 'got ahead' she might have been one of the only women at the table so she had to learn to be competitive to climb the ladder, which I empathise with. But I don't think younger women feel that way as much. We didn't enter the workplace feeling like we needed to elbow other women out of the way. At the end of the day, good work is born out of collaboration.

I have often felt that resentment, that things were perhaps 'harder' when I started off in my career, and I have thought that younger women have it easier. However, the truth is that the context has shifted and things aren't necessarily easier – they're just different. Certainly, the amount of work that's expected from the average person has hiked up significantly, with every minute of every day expected to be productive. Whatever has changed, there are still things you can bring to the table that your younger colleagues can't – there are also lots of things you can learn from them. Recently I was working on an online platform for research and it was making me paranoid because I couldn't quite get the hang of it. So, I texted a younger colleague and asked her to help. It took her ten minutes to walk me through it all, and in return I talked her through some interviewing techniques. Previously I would have just felt grumpy and out of the loop and defensive (and pretended I knew what I was doing because I wanted to preserve the sense of hierarchy) but instead I felt like we both learnt something. We weren't competing either. We were supporting one another and making life easier.

Maybe there is no such thing as a DREAM job

I wish someone had told me early on that not everyone finds their ultimate, amazing, most fabulous, BEST JOB EVER job – the thing that they jump out of bed in the morning and shout 'HALLELUJAH!' because they're so excited to be doing it. My unhappiness about my job in the past has essentially stemmed from two things: my innate sense of insecurity and imposter syndrome, and the fact that I kept thinking that somewhere there was a job that was far better suited to me. There probably was one somewhere, but I have no clear idea of what it might have been.

I'm forty-seven now and still don't really know what job I want to do. I love writing. I enjoy talking to people. I love finding out weird things about human behaviour. I'm curious. I've now realised that it's okay to have a day job that I don't always find amazing and fulfilling. The truth is that many of us have to work in order to survive, and for me (as the breadwinner) I can't afford to pursue a job that makes me happy (my partner can't just rent me an art gallery as an interesting side project).

The pressure for the job to be amazing is too much. (This doesn't mean you can't dream; just don't feel crap if it's not your reality right now – the bills need to be paid, right?)

Sometimes when I look on social media, I get the impression that everyone is doing something vastly more interesting than me, but this isn't the whole truth. Yes, there are some people who make a decent living from being influencers and gadding about at events, but many others have regular jobs – jobs that provide the stability they need to live normal lives and not sit up at night worrying about finances.

Skill-swapping and job-sharing

I'm good at people stuff – managing difficult personalities, calming shit down when people aren't getting on, and making interactions on teams run smoothly. These are all important skills. However, I'm not good with figures and pie charts and data and percentages – I find my brain zones out.

One of the benefits of age is knowing what you're good at and realising that you can't be good at everything. Like I said earlier, there is no shame in asking for help or learning from a younger colleague – in fact, it's a really good idea.

Emma Gannon echoes this point:

> I love the idea of skill-swapping and also job-sharing. In my book I share an example of job-sharing that works really well, allowing both people a stable regular income and giving them free time on the side to grow their own projects. This in turn makes them more money than a 9–5 salary. I think it's a good thing to do, regardless of age, as we all have different super powers. I also love seeing a life-skill swap in action whenever I interview anyone in their seventies or eighties. I've taught them how to make a podcast, and they've told me unforgettable wisdom on how to set boundaries, say no and give less of a shit :-)

Role models are important

Many of the older women I worked with weren't aspirational. The adage is *we can't be what we can't see*. Many of the boss women I saw when I was moving up the ranks were unsympathetic and hard and seemed to favour men or women who acted like men. This wasn't entirely their fault. They'd adapted to get ahead – if you wanted to be a boss in the 90s, then you copied the men around you and adopted their values. Some wore giant shoulder pads in order to assert their alpha female-ness. I once got told off by my boss for drinking a pint of beer (this was when beer was all the rage but there was this weird dichotomy where women were expected to have power bobs and masculine clothes but then sip on white wine and laugh at men's jokes).

Others seemed to have had their empathy surgically removed and had turned themselves into robots. Some were incredibly sexist and didn't believe that motherhood and work were compatible. All this shaped the company culture and made it permissible to say certain offensive things and get away with it. Now, thankfully, work is changing and there are more role models (but still not enough). Even if you're in your forties or fifties, it can be good to have role models – women doing work that you respect, in a company culture that is progressive and modern, with empathy and people skills at the core.

It's also never too late to get a mentor. You might even consider a younger mentor. Nobody dictates the age they should be and I'm increasingly finding that younger people inspire me (as long as I stop getting jealous of their glowing skin).

Keep learning and adapting

Annie Auerbach admits that, yes, there is ageism in the workplace, *but* there are tactics we can use to give ourselves an advantage:

> We live in a very ageist society, but women suffer from ageism more than men, as society equates their power to appearance. Older people, particularly women, are airbrushed out of society, and out of culture – women cite 'invisibility' as being a consequence of ageing. We need to move towards being proud of our ages and writing ourselves back into the script.

She also believes that age is a good thing when it comes to work, but we've been educated to feel it isn't, which results in massive insecurity:

> With age comes experience, expertise, the ability to relax into situations which we've seen and dealt with before, the ability to empathise with others earlier on in their careers. If you are a mum, dominant work culture might have duped you into thinking that that is a weakness. But being a parent is a superpower in the workforce – you are resilient, adaptable, a problem solver and a lateral thinker.

Annie also believes that staying abreast of technology and updating your work skills is important:

> My advice would be that tech is changing so rapidly that everyone has to learn and relearn throughout their careers. Don't see yourself as on the 'backfoot' – the pace of change affects everyone. Find ways to incorporate learning and new skills into your life; see education as a lifelong thing rather than something you front load your life with.

Say what you think and don't hold back

Sometimes it's okay if you're difficult. Sometimes it's okay to say the thing that everyone else is thinking. You have a right to your opinion and you have the experience behind you to know what you're talking about. You're not just shooting crap in the wind. Remember that your older male colleagues won't be pissing themselves in fear about that important meeting. Instead they'll be listening to Bon Jovi in the car and getting ready to NAIL IT with some flippant comment they read on the back of Richard Branson's autobiography.

I sat through so many meetings and was quiet, too scared to say the wrong thing. I witnessed men half my age saying the wrong thing and getting away with it because they were seen as geniuses. There was one guy I worked with who did a loud burp in a high-profile client meeting and everyone laughed (I felt that if I'd done this, I wouldn't have received the same reaction). After one long meeting (I was a Managing Partner at this stage), one of my colleagues said, 'Well, what do you think, Anniki? Please do offer us your wisdom.' And I couldn't think of one single comment to add. I was struck dumb. It is only now, six years later, that I realise I was so insecure about my own opinion, so worried that I'd get it wrong, that I thought it was best to say nothing at all. This obviously doesn't make you very memorable long term.

Annie puts it best:

> Having a bold opinion is gold dust. If I look back on my career, I always self-censored and silenced myself, and the joy of it when you get older is saying what you think and shedding all that baggage.

If you're in your forties and can't say what you REALLY think, then when can you?

Do things you love but don't feel like you need to have a side hustle just because everyone else does

I used to get severe anxiety whenever anyone mentioned the words 'SIDE HUSTLE'. I'd be at influencer events, feeling like a blobby-no-mates and then someone would sidle up to me and say, 'Hey, what's your side hustle, hun?' and I'd get anxiety. It felt like *another* thing to worry about (as well as being a parent, having a job/a nice house/a good relationship/five million followers). Basically, a side hustle is the new buzz word for 'HOBBY'. Our grans would have done *Arrow* word puzzles or made those crochet things you put on the corner of chairs. They would have baked cakes or grown enormous courgettes. Of course, there are some side hustles that turn into businesses but many are just hobbies and that's fine. No pressure. There's been a lot of stuff written about 'side hustles' and sometimes it feels like another pressure for the older woman to take on board (i.e. I have to bring up kids, have fulfilling work, be fit, have a great sex life and also develop a whole sideline that will turn into a business, which will mean I can give up my day job and do the thing I really love forever).

I have met lots of women with side hustles and many of them love having something that they feel passionate about (and this is great, especially when you're ageing and can feel stuck), *but* the majority of side hustles won't earn you a fortune or allow you to give up your day job. I've discovered that many of the women I thought were earning a fortune from side hustles had two things in common: a) they were already loaded or b) had rich husbands.

I beat myself up for a long time about being unable to make my side hustle produce enough money to support my family *until* I realised that there is only really a minority of women who do this. Most have to work in jobs. Normal jobs. Not jobs that you read about in magazines which are highly glamorous and dynamic and involve a treadmill desk and a direct line to Anna Wintour.

Don't undersell yourself – nobody is going to sell you for you

After I'd had my second daughter I returned to market research. I'd previously managed an entire company but now felt out of the loop. Washed up. No good work vibes. There was part of me that didn't want the level of responsibility that I'd had before I had kids. I took on a role and it was way more junior than the one I'd had before. I felt that I needed to apologise for wanting to work part-time and didn't deserve a big job with a big salary. I was a mum. I was old. Who would consider me an asset? Even right now I'm applying for jobs that are below my pay-grade. I am not good at selling myself. On the one hand there's no shame in wanting to opt out of the big shoulder-padded top-dog jobs because you want to combine your work with other things, but don't put yourself down (this is clearly advice I need to take myself too).

Don't be scared to call out bad behaviour

When I was younger there were lots of examples of behaviours that were sexist and ageist (comments about younger female colleagues and how shaggable they were). This was before #metoo and the climate of openness that we live in now (which still has a way to go but is definitely more progressive than it was fifteen years ago). Now I'm more likely to say something if someone says something sexist in a meeting. I'm less worried about what others think and less willing to put up with bad behaviour. Recently I was talking to a male colleague and I told him I was passionate about seeing more women on the boards of companies and it was something I'd written about and had chaired an event about.

'Oh well in my experience that's not a problem,' he said casually. 'I mean it used to be but not anymore.'

He puffed up his chest and looked at me with a superior air. In the past I would have sucked this up and apologised for his bullshit, but now the more outspoken side won't tolerate macho nonsense.

'Well it's hardly surprising!' I said. 'You're a man! You wouldn't have experienced any problems anyway. You're not the expert, are you?'

He looked at me and was obviously put out. In the old days I would have then felt guilty about making him feel awkward and I would have analysed the situation and thought about how I could ease his discomfort by pretending that, yes, he was a bigger feminist than I was and he was RIGHT. Just like you should aim to say something in meetings, you should definitely call time on negative stereotypes – sexism, racism, ageism, sizeism – the whole caboodle. This isn't about age but is more about just fighting inequality. I love women who come out and say exactly what they think. I am working to be more like them.

Fuck the work drinks (unless you love the work drinks)

One of the worst things that has come out of the 24/7 work culture has been the notion that you need to socialise with your colleagues as well as spend all your days chained to a desk with them. I really feel that by the time you reach your forties you are allowed to sack the work drinks off (unless you want to escape your family and are actually looking forward to the work drinks because they're in a nice bar in Shoreditch and you rarely get the opportunity to go out anymore).

It's okay to take your foot off the accelerator

Depending on your circumstances, you may find that you haven't got the passion for work that you had in your twenties or early thirties. You might not have the energy either. That's okay. Work is work, and the endless pursuit of trying to find THE JOB THAT CHANGES YOUR LIFE is exhausting. Working for promotions and travelling and always saying 'yes' is also knackering. There are times in life when it makes sense to really focus on your career, and there are times when it is simply too much and you might just want to coast along without thinking too much about it. I worked in McDonalds for three years when I was in my teens. I am under no illusion that it was hard work and knackering, but there was something okay about coming into work and going home without emails arriving at 10pm or sleepless nights worrying about whether the Zoom meeting connection would be okay (is this the new anxiety when we're working from home?). I worked in retail and had a similar experience – but I appreciate you can still have politics and crap management wherever you are. I'm not being romantic about tough jobs, especially if they're tiring, poorly paid ones, but back then I needed a job that demanded little from me.

I have now reached the stage where I want work that ticks lots of different boxes, and that makes things trickier. I also have to balance making money with doing what I love. Eventually I'll move to a position where making money and the things I love come together in a beautiful union.

This will take time.

In the meantime, don't let the bastards get you down, remember to stop the negative chatter in its tracks and remember that no bad situation lasts forever.

**Five things to say in meetings to show
your enthusiasm and demonstrate that you care**

1. 'That's really interesting.' I have built my entire career on
   this. I use the word 'interesting' about a hundred times a
   day and it never gets old (unlike myself).
2. Quote a stat that you've read about the category/product/
   topic you're talking about. I knew a male colleague who
   always had a stat that he'd researched before he went into
   meetings – it really works as long as you GET IT RIGHT.
   Otherwise, it will bite you in the ass.
3. Say something newsworthy (i.e. that shows that you know
   what's going on in the world and how it relates to what
   you're talking about) but avoid politics if it's a work meeting.
   So, you could say, 'I heard that sales of garden furniture
   are really going up as people are spending an increasing
   amount of time in their gardens this year.' But don't say, 'I
   think Donald Trump would like your product as he's rather
   challenged in the hair department.'
4. Say, 'Does anyone want a cup of tea/drink?' Again, this
   is frowned upon, but I firmly believe that if people are
   thirsty, they get fed up, the meeting dynamic is awful and
   ultimately the meeting won't be successful. I've sat through
   epic meetings where the sandwiches were stale because they'd
   sat uncovered for too long, the tea had gone cold, there was
   no coffee in the urn and everyone was despondent. In one
   simple move I would get some refreshments and suddenly
   the mood would swing up again. They'd usually give credit

to the guy who was quoting some bollocks about Baudelaire, but it was ME all along who had shifted the bad energy.

5. Make some small talk but don't be too revealing. This is something I struggle with a lot as I am generally an over-sharer. I have walked into a meeting and told people I have my period. I have also told a client that I had a relative who committed suicide. This is not professional and it is why I am not the head of my own company and worth millions of pounds. Yes, there is a role to connect through shared vulnerability, as Brené Brown argues in her brilliant books and podcasts, but there's a time and a place for it. It's best when you first meet someone and it's business time (and not the *Flight of the Conchords* kind of business time) to just keep things light: 'How was your journey?' 'The weather is nice, right?' 'I, too, have a dog, and he likes walks.'

… That kind of thing.

What is a side hustle?

I've already touched on the concept of a side hustle (i.e. *a hobby*), but whenever I hear those words I think of that disco dance where people used to turn around and clap their hands in the air and there was a flute playing in the background. I can hear it even now (the song is called 'Do the Hustle', apparently).

It turns my stomach because it has become a bit of a cliché and seems to be another THING that women are expected to accomplish before they clamber into their wicker coffin and take the longest nap known to womankind.

Who invented the term? And can they please shut up about it? (I looked it up and actually the term has been around since the 1950s so isn't as new as we think.)

The first definition when I type 'what is a side hustle' into Google reads thus:

> A **side hustle** is any type of employment undertaken in addition to one's full-time job. A **side hustle** is generally freelance or piecework in nature, providing a supplemental income. **Side hustles** are often things a person is passionate about, rather than a typical day job worked in order to make ends meet.

Side hustles are great if you're dipping your toe in the water to see if you want to do a particular thing. They can help restore self-esteem and identity after you've had kids and feel like your head is a marshmallow full of sludgy wet-wipes. They can be the first rung of a new business. They could be a way to earn extra dosh.

For ten years my side hustle has been writing.

I would say that writing is still my side hustle because I'll be honest and say it doesn't provide enough income to support my family. I continue to work day jobs which pay the bills whilst the writing ticks away until one day I'll explode and become the kind of writer who has her own proper office and gets asked to literary festivals and makes a decent enough living to give it her whole focus.

'I'm not really sure what my side hustle would be if I had one,' a friend said to me recently. 'I'm teaching full-time, have two young kids and barely have the time to keep the house in order, let alone develop a passion project.'

'Well maybe you don't have one right now. Maybe you don't have one at all. That's fine, right?' I replied.

'But everyone else has a podcast or a book or a business idea and I feel really boring,' she replied.

And that's the thing with side hustles: IT'S ACTUALLY OKAY IF YOU DON'T HAVE ONE BECAUSE YOU HAVE TOO MUCH OTHER STUFF TO DO AND HAVE TO WORK TO

EARN MONEY EACH DAY/HAVE KIDS TO LOOK AFTER/
ELDERLY RELATIVES/WHATEVER IT IS THAT EATS UP
ALL YOUR TIME.

It somehow feels to me like having one of these things is compulsory. The modern side hustle of course (in Instagram circles) is the podcast. Podcasts are fab and great and I absolutely love them and I have one myself. *However*, you can be a successful, functioning woman and *not* have a podcast. You can be a successful, functioning woman and *not* have a clothing line. Or an online store. Or a business making vitamin supplements for cats. I sometimes look at the number of podcasts and feel like there is actually NO POINT in me having one because there are so many fascinating, interesting perspectives and why would anyone want to listen to me anyway?

I think aliens are looking down on us right now, and aside from being freaked out that we're all wearing masks and trying to social distance, they'll say:

'What are these damn podcast things? They seem to be all over the place.'

'Apparently every human needs to have one. If you don't have one, then you're not seen as successful.'

'But what are they all talking about and why won't they stop?'

And then the alien slithers away with his iPhone under his tentacle and his wireless headphones on, secretly listening to Adam Buxton and actually quite enjoying it (this is my favourite podcast and I don't mind if he continues to make a hundred of them).

Take the pressure off yourself okay?

I love having a passion in my life and having dreams. I don't love the constant expectation that I will support my family from my passion. I've spoken to many amazing women who are pursuing their dreams, and the majority of them are struggling to make ends meet. A lot of stuff you do in the name of the side hustle is done for free. Things are often phrased as 'good for your profile' and so you get asked to do something like write some FREE CONTENT or attend an event and TALK FOR TWO HOURS ABOUT HOW TO HAVE A SUCCESSFUL SIDE HUSTLE. Some people can afford to do this, but the majority can't.

As we get older it's okay to realise that actually you can only do a certain amount each day and that sitting in a chair and staring at a wall is just as useful and helpful to your mental wellbeing as trying to edit a podcast or write a memoir or kickstart your beanie hat for pugs business.

Even the term 'hustle' makes me feel exhausted – as if you're constantly going up to people and trying to play them and are always looking out for opportunities to further yourself and get a selfie with a big influencer so you can increase your profile. A hobby is old-fashioned perhaps, but it implies you can pick it up and put it down whenever you like… and it's relaxing. You may go on to make a lot of money from it but you may just use it to get more enjoyment out of life. My mum loves embroidery and knits like mad. She can even make those macramé plant basket things that are in every designer influencer feed I click on. She enjoys doing this stuff but she doesn't put the pressure on herself to launch it as a business. It's a hobby. It's relaxing. It's okay to leave it that way.

If you want to start your own business, then that's another thing. Let's not call it a side hustle. Let's call it a business as that's what it is, with all the associated risks and pitfalls. I spoke to Molly Gunn who's the founder of Selfish Mother. Selfish Mother was a blog to begin with, providing a forum for hundreds of women to write about their experiences of motherhood. It then evolved into a clothing line with distinctive slogan sweatshirts (with impressive amounts of the business proceeds going to charity). I used to work for Molly and edited the Selfish Mother blog for a couple of years.

It helped me develop my writing as I regularly posted short articles. I then felt chuffed when they resonated and this encouraged me to keep at it. I wanted to better understand how she'd gone about launching the business (i.e. the reality rather than the fantasy).

Molly started the business whilst she was on maternity leave. Initially, she had no idea how it would end up:

> It started as a blog in 2013 and didn't make any money for the first year, so I just edited it in my evenings. I was a freelance journalist by day, and then also worked on my husband's T-shirt business, Millionhands. One day I asked him to design a tee for me that said 'MOTHER' and I launched one hundred of them to my blog audience to raise money for Women for Women International… They sold out in twenty-four hours! That was July 2014… About six months later I was running Selfish Mother as my full-time job.

She didn't have lots of cash to invest in the business and so she started out small: 'I didn't invest in it or have any savings! I simply ordered small quantities of tees and paid for them as I sold them.' She knew the business had potential but didn't know how it would ultimately net out: 'I knew my husband had succeeded with selling his T-shirts, but I didn't know it would work for Selfish Mother… I am stoked to still be selling tees six years later.'

If you are starting a business, then you may have to combine working on your day job and starting up your business, especially if you're dependent on your day job income. Molly's advice is:

> Don't give up everything immediately. Also, don't tell everyone what you are up to as sometimes people don't 'get' your idea and they kind of put you off it (without meaning to)… Only share your vision with people you think will be supportive and really 'get it', or at least pretend to!

Now that Molly has her own business, she doesn't want to go back to working for someone else. However, she does acknowledge the fact that combining a day job with your own business can have certain attractions and advantages. She says:

> If I lived in London I might [work for someone else] as day jobs might be more flexible these days... but Bruton would be too far of a commute! I would quite like someone else to pay me! I used to love going to work and getting all dressed up and feeling all snazzy working in fashion journalism, but I do quite like running my own biz and working whenever I want to.

So, side hustles are one thing, but don't feel like you have to HUSTLE 24/7 and have some productive passion project in order to be accepted as a fully paid-up member of the forty-something superwoman club.

Starting a business is not easy either and it's worth being mindful of what's sending you down that route in the first place.

I find that the times when I'm most miserable at work are the times when I fantasise most about starting my own business. So far I've *almost* launched an app that delivers risotto straight to your door and nearly started an ice-cream parlour that serves flavours named after famous rock stars. Luckily I never pursued any of these ideas, but if there is already someone doing these things, GOOD LUCK to them!

(And, yes, I believe there is a future in personalised alpaca baby hats, even if nobody else does, okay?)

Top ten things to do when you feel old and shit

1. Put 90s music on and dance.
2. Have a bath with essential oils and put some hair removal cream on your chin/lip/sideburns.
3. Listen to one of Nora Ephron's audio books (anything by Nora Ephron will be soothing).
4. Watch *St Elmo's Fire* and marvel at the fact that Demi Moore looks younger today than she did in 1985.
5. Masturbate.
6. Dig out the old packet of cigarettes that live in your knicker drawer, wait till the children are in bed and smoke one in the garden, imagining you are in a French film and your lover is just about to seduce you and then take you for a midnight motorcycle ride around Paris.
7. Go swimming (ideally in a river/the sea if you can).
8. Phone an old friend and complain about how old you feel right now.
9. Don't watch TikTok or feel compelled to make a TikTok video – you'll look like a twat.
10. Exercise.

Why I grew up thinking older women were scary motherfuckers

When I was growing up I was a massive TV and film addict, like most kids growing up in the 80s. I loved nothing more than sitting about two inches away from the TV (the picture was crap and we had to manually change the station and fiddle with the aerial to get a clear visual). In terms of films, I had a few firm favourites. There was *The Goonies*. Then the Disney classics like *Snow White* and *Cinderella* and *101 Dalmatians*. Then *The Wizard of Oz*, which was terrifying of course. Then there was reading – and I did a lot of reading of books like *Rapunzel* and *Hansel & Gretel*. Or Roald Dahl's *The Witches* (I loved Roald Dahl and read all of his books obsessively before moving onto Judy Blume in my early teens).

It's only now that I realise that many of these narratives had old women in pivotal roles. These old women were remarkably similar. *They were evil witches who liked harming children.*

Think about the female crook in *The Goonies* (played by actress Angelina Ramsey, who specialised in evil old ladies). This woman is so cruel and frightening that she threatens to put Chunk's hand in a food blender. I imagine there are many female media students who have written essays about the depictions of women in Disney films (all those passive princesses waiting to be saved by dashing, forceful young men) but the older women in these films are more depressing (usually ugly, bitter, hateful, mean, and jealous of young women and their beauty). I loved *The Witches*, but the women in that film are basically monsters who disguise themselves with masks so they can plan how to kill children and take over the world. Then there's *Tangled*, with the horrible witch controlling Rapunzel's powers so she can be eternally youthful. Now that I've grown older, I've realised the depiction of older women when I was growing up was shit.

Some of this is just for dramatic intent. It's fun to watch an evil baddie and be scared and cower behind the sofa, but there definitely isn't a sense that growing older as a woman is something to celebrate. Instead, I thought when you got old you'd be depressed and isolated (although maybe not resorting to eating kids).

I still struggle to think of kids' films that represent old women in a positive way. I loved *Up* because of its depiction of an old man and the way he refuses to back down to authority when a big building corporation wants to knock down his beloved home. I also loved *The Little Prince* because it had a fantastic male character that reminded me of my dad and made me cry quite a lot. There are more feisty, aspirational girls in Disney films now: *Inside Out*, *Frozen* (sort of), *Brave*. And what about teaching young girls about what ageing will look like for them? *What if we don't want to grow up and be a witch? (And is it surprising that there still lurks the stereotype of the grumpy, old, abandoned woman who lives alone with cats.)*

And is it strange that when I got into my forties I started to feel a bit depressed at the prospect of old age? Can you think of any older positive female role models in Disney films? So far I've got the granny in *Moana* but not much else. (Answers on a postcard please.)

CHAPTER SIX

Moods, Hump Days, Hormones and Menopause

Aside from not learning enough about waning fertility at school, there was also zero mention of the menopause. There might have been the odd reference to 'hot flushes' in teatime TV sitcoms, but once I got into my mid-forties, I felt ill-prepared for the hormonal fluctuations I experienced. I was lucky enough to have recorded a podcast for *The Hotbed* and interviewed Meg Mathews, who was very open about her own struggles with the menopause. She'd been unaware that the lack of energy and pain she was feeling were symptoms and so thought she had arthritis. So, I started thinking that some of the physical and emotional junk I was going through weren't just sleep deprivation because of a new baby. I felt like even on the nights I wasn't getting woken my children, I was still sleeping poorly – possibly because I was starting to see the beginning of peri-menopause which can mess up your sleeping patterns too of course.

What's the menopause? (You probably know this part already, but just in case you don't...)

The menopause is when your periods stop and you are no longer able to get pregnant naturally. This is usually a gradual process, with periods becoming less frequent in the lead-up (peri-menopause). Sometimes, though, they can stop suddenly with little or no warning. The menopause usually happens when a woman is between the ages of forty-five and fifty-five, but 1:100 women will experience menopause before the age of forty. This is known as 'premature menopause' or 'premature ovarian insufficiency'.

Common symptoms of the peri-menopause and menopause include:

- hot flushes
- night sweats
- vaginal dryness (which can make sex uncomfortable)
- difficulty sleeping
- a muddled or foggy brain
- anxiety
- low mood or depression
- loss of libido or low libido.

If you sit in a room with women who are all going through it, then it's likely that you'll be experiencing different stuff. Some women have bonkers night sweats. Others are plagued by pins and needles. There can also be heavy emotional side to it, with feelings of sadness, loss, depression and anxiety suddenly rising to the surface. There is quite a lot of fear around the peri-menopause and menopause. In my survey, women worried about what kind of symptoms they might have and how they'd cope when the time came. (It was a bit like that phrase in *Game of Thrones* where they kept saying 'winter is coming' – nobody quite knew what that winter meant, but it was likely to be bad.)

I'm not looking forward to the physical side of menopause. I worry that it will hit me hard.

I look forward to being post-menopausal but dread [the actual menopause] happening.

I'm scared that my body is about to fail me.

I didn't pick up any feedback from women who were looking forward to the menopause or saw much of a silver lining associated with it. This is sad as it's something we're all going to go through, and whilst it may bring some challenges, the more fear we have, the more difficult it's going to feel. It's like those days when you get up and say to yourself, 'Today's going to be a shitstorm of a day.' And what happens? It's a dreadful day, right? I'm not saying you should prance about like a Disney character singing a merry tune (but it would be interesting to have a Disney character who displayed symptoms of the menopause because that might normalise it) but if it's going to happen, then let's at least feel prepared for what comes, talk about it and seek help if necessary.

In terms of my own personal experience, I'm not yet perimenopausal. It turns out that the symptoms I was getting (and am still getting) are related to having a baby in my mid-forties. It's given me a good 'menopause taster session' (but who really wants one?) as I've had night sweats and woken up regularly with my hair stuck to my neck and needing to change my T-shirt and get fresh bed sheets out. I've had rabid anxiety – this started six months after my daughter was born – and became so feverish that I had to see an NHS counsellor and have Cognitive Behaviour Therapy (CBT) to help me look at things more clearly. I'll look at anxiety in more detail in the next chapter as these are anxious times and it seems that everyone I speak to is suffering from it (understandably, with all the shit that's going down, i.e. A GLOBAL PANDEMIC). Today my anxiety is not so bad but tomorrow it might come back first thing (for me it's always worse in the mornings). I can be perfectly okay one minute and the next get butterflies in my stomach and a strong sense of impending doom. I've learnt coping strategies, and the counselling helped, but usually the bouts will last an hour or two and then pass. They're particularly bad if I've had a couple of drinks the night before or too much caffeine.

The kind of thoughts that go through my head when I'm anxious are:

> *I'm a shit parent.*
> *I haven't achieved anywhere near what I want to achieve.*
> *Time is running out.*
> *I have a beard.*
> *I hate my body.*
> *I hate my life.*
> *I have no real friends.*
> *I am going to be destitute because I won't find another job.*
> *Nobody will hire me because I'm too old.*
> *I have a beard like Kenny Rodgers and it seems to be getting longer each day.*

(The beard one is usually on a loop and comes back every hour or so, no matter how bad my anxiety is that day.)

The other thing that people don't talk about much is ANGER (which I touched on earlier because we need to talk about it). Women can be quite scared by anger as we're brought up to push unpleasant emotions under the surface, but I've noticed a lot more anger as I've moved past my mid-forties. I'm still getting my period, and the days leading up to it are usually pretty bad anger-wise. For example:

- As already mentioned, I like to throw things out of the window.
- I like to sulk and then expect my family to guess what's up with me. And then I get very worked up when nobody actually notices that I'm sulking (i.e. I haven't said anything all day long and nobody actually cares).

- If I'm not sulking, then I rant. Anything can set off a rant, but it will usually be some domestic stuff that hasn't been done – for example, it could be that there is no toilet roll in the loo despite there being toilet roll in the cupboard (I get really angry when someone leaves a little cardboard roll with no paper but can't be arsed to pick the toilet roll up from next to the loo and replace it).

I know that there are massive injustices going on in the world. I get angry about these things too. I wish I could do something about all these injustices (and on a good day I try) but I find that the anger I go through when I'm hormonal is very unhelpful. I have to just ride it out. It eventually subsides but it isn't the kind that inspires me to do useful things. I tend to say hurtful stuff. I shout. I break things. It's ugly.

Menopause is complicated. Some women laugh it off and say they're looking forward to not getting periods anymore. Or they just fan their faces and say it's getting a bit hot. However, in a culture where we sometimes deny ageing is happening, where everyone looks so youthful and is still keeping up demanding schedules and trying to achieve stuff, menopause feels like a reality check:

> *Think you're still young because you've made a TikTok dance routine? Well, here comes a night sweat baby! You're getting the menopause. You can't hide! It doesn't matter how fresh your trainers are or whether you've dyed your hair rose gold – the menopause is coming for ya!*

It would be easy to sink into depression if you didn't really know what was happening to your body. Looking through my survey, the following quote really jumped out in summarising the isolation many women feel during menopause and also how society treats the whole experience as a 'bit of a laugh':

I feel utterly useless. My mind feels like I'm underwater most of the time. Although I opened up to female colleagues, they used it against me. They made fun of my constant, muddled mind. So much so, I cried on the way home. I feel less relevant in the world, in my home, at the school gates, and it is a very scary time.

Sam Baker, author of *The Shift: How I (lost and) found myself after 40 – and you can too*, said: 'I thought I was going mad. I am a woman used to using words for a living but I'd lost the power of words. My brain was muddled.' Comments like these are shocking because menopause is something we all go through and yet women are still feeling isolated and ridiculed when they fess up to it (when they're most in need of connection and sympathy).

Celebrities have spoken about the emotional impact of menopause. Lorraine Kelly said:

I couldn't understand why I felt flat. There was no reason for it. I wasn't depressed exactly, but there was a sense of not seeing the joy in anything. I'd lost my mojo… and I was tired. Bone tired. I couldn't understand it. (Interview in the *Daily Mail*, 22 September 2017)

And Ulrika Jonsson said:

Depression has been a regular feature of my life, and then came the most unimaginable anxiety that I've not known before. Anxiety like proper panic – at one stage I thought my head was going to explode. (Interview on *Lorraine* TV show, 6 October 2017)

I tend to plunge into negative thought patterns at times and so once I get into the menopause for real, I worry that I too will descend into darkness. The main thing, however, is being prepared for these feelings. I know that if I'm prepared then I can use some of the things in my tool box to dig me out again (more about these in the anxiety chapter).

Karen Arthur is a fashion designer, blogger, public speaker, founder of 'Wear Your Happy' and teaches sewing. She has been through the menopause and I wanted to talk to her because she's on a mission to bring menopause out of the closet. Her mindset is incredibly positive and part of that stems from the fact that she talks about it, accepts it's happened and has found tools and survival mechanisms that work for her. She very much felt that the menopause had taken her by surprise:

> I didn't have a clue. I suddenly had the house to myself because the children had left home. I was fifty-two and I thought I'd love having the place to myself but instead I felt lonely and kept on wanting to call British Gas. When I went to the GP, we talked about my depression and my work but we didn't really talk about the menopause.

The emotional impact of the menopause is massive and tends to make you feel like you're invisible. So, it's important not to minimise what you're going through. It is a significant change and society hasn't really caught up with the idea that women are going through a challenging time and need support and empathy.

The fact that depression could be a symptom of the menopause was new to me. This is often the challenge with the peri-menopause and menopause. It doesn't visit us when we're having nice restful lives and we can give all our attention to it. It arrives when we're in the rush hour of life – with or without kids, working, dealing with our new identities, our changing bodies/faces and trying to figure out what the future is going to look like.

Karen felt that ultimately the menopause gave her the insight that she needed to seize the day and make the most of the life she had left: 'I then suffered a bereavement and my eldest daughter wasn't well; and the thing is, of course, we're getting older and of course we're going to die. It doesn't have to be depressing though.' These things, and the arrival of the menopause, made Karen realise that she had to focus more on the present: 'I realise now that we need to live for the present. I am having a great time because I'm allowing life to do what it does. I'm not trying to control everything anymore.'

Part of dealing with menopause is facing up to our own mortality. This can obviously be very frightening but it also helps to throw things into perspective. It ultimately reminds us that time spent hiding our light behind a bushel is wasted time.

What about work and the menopause?

Interestingly, it seems a fairly common theme that women who hit the menopause have a massive re-think about their lives and can hopefully use this momentum to pivot into a new direction. However, there are also those who stay in the same roles at work, feeling more and more invisible and unloved, or struggling to find a job because they lack self-belief and feel like they haven't got the skills to take on the modern world of work. On the one hand you SHOULD have confidence. This is what we see in the typical advertising campaigns aimed at older women: sassy, dominant, women who have reached a stage of not caring what others think and so can happily embrace their true identities, whilst wearing high-tech incontinence pads or the latest anti-ageing face creams. The truth is that you don't just arrive at that stage without going through the not-feeling-so-great phase first (or the majority of us don't). It's like you're in the jungle and you're chopping back the shame, the tiredness, the sense of irrelevancy, the night sweats, and you're learning how to deal with these things and falling over because your foot has got caught in a massive tree root; eventually, you emerge into a bit of a clearing which leads to a beach and the ocean and that's when you get to prance about perhaps ('prance' might not be the right word here – it might be more of a limp).

So, when it comes to work, now may not be the right time to do this pivoting thing. Instead, it may be the right time to focus on being kind to yourself and getting through your current job or finding something that 'works for now' and gradually building up a picture through writing things down and talking to friends about what you want your work life to look like. When I was stuck, finding a life coach helped (see the previous chapter on the benefit of getting a coach – there are ones who focus specifically on work). Life coaching can be pricey, depending on who you choose, but I worked with my coach because I genuinely felt lost in terms of my work life. I wanted to move away from market research, which was what I'd done for years, and do more of the things that I loved, but this had to work financially. She helped me see things a bit more clearly – like I've said already, I'm not currently going through the peri-menopause but I'm still experiencing brain fug, lack of clarity and anxiety, and so trying to get a plan together in terms of work felt like an impossible task. I was, and still am some days, stuck in the jungle with no tools to chop anything down, making zero progress forward, with the beach and the opportunity to prance about on it seemingly impossible to reach. Just knowing that the beach is there is reassuring and I've got more tools at my disposal to reach that place eventually. (I'll stop with the jungle analogy now, okay?)

There are things we can do to help ourselves and we don't have to suffer on our own. Nowadays there is less of a taboo associated with the menopause and there are an increasing number of books and podcasts being launched that talk openly about the challenges. One of the key things is to not ignore the symptoms. Do some research (I have provided a list of resources at the end of the book) and speak to your GP.

Karen explored a few different things, and combined together they helped her feel better both mentally and physically:

I finally had therapy which was the best gift I've ever given myself. Therapy is expensive and I was lucky in that I could afford to have it. As a Black woman, I wanted another Black woman. I only left the house to go to therapy. I discovered mindful meditation. I got silent and went from a really stressful job and going to school and checking emails to nothing. I had to get silent.

She also believes that our culture of always being busy masks what's going on inside and so believes we need to slow down and take time to think about what we want for the next phase of our life:

We spend too much time championing the busy, and life doesn't have to be so busy and difficult. The times when I've had the luxury to sit and go slowly is when the answers come. I also discovered my love of fashion. Clothes were a massive deal for me. Wearing things that I love, like colour or a bright head wrap, and I love posh lingerie and lovely textures. Vintage clothing, too. Clothing and meeting up with people going through the same thing as me have helped massively.

Despite more women opening up about the menopause, if you are a menopausal woman of colour there's a real dearth of women to look to for guidance and advice. Women like Karen are brilliant because they are sharing their experience and can hopefully provide a platform for more women of colour to share theirs. She believes this is because society as a whole judges menopausal women as being pretty much pointless:

We don't celebrate getting older in women. If you talk about menopause, then people know you're older, and you're outed. Judi Dench on the cover of *Vogue* – that's celebrated as groundbreaking when it shouldn't be groundbreaking. I stopped dying my hair because I was fed up of being told by advertisers that dying my

hair would reveal the real me. I am the real me with my silver hair!
I have earned every strand.

Karen is on a mission to rebalance the representation of
women and the menopause with a specific focus on increasing
diversity, which is much needed. This means seeing not only
more women of different ages in the media but also seeing
women from different ethnic backgrounds. If you think it's crap
for white women, then wait until you try and seek out more
diverse, older female role models. Karen says, 'Where are the
role models that champion menopausal women? And if we look
at Black women, we have Angela Bassett in the U.S. maybe, but
that's for her young looks.'

Managing the Menopause

One of the most useful women I've turned to in preparation for
the menopause is 'The Menopause Doctor', Dr Louise R, Newson
who is a GP, Menopause Specialist and founder of The Menopause
Charity. I've summarised some of the key information she provides,
but check out her website for more info (see Resources section).

What's HRT? The basics

One of the most effective treatments for the menopause is to replace
the hormones that your body is no longer producing. Hormone
Replacement Therapy (HRT) includes the hormones oestrogen,
often progestogen (a medication that produces similar effects to
progesterone), and sometimes testosterone. It also has some health
benefits (it lowers the risks of developing heart disease, osteoporosis,
diabetes, depression and dementia), but you still need to take care
of yourself in terms of getting regular exercise, eating healthy food
and cutting back on booze.

What are the risks?

For most women the benefits of taking HRT outweigh any risks (if you're under sixty when you start taking it). There are, however, a couple of risks: the risk of breast cancer and the risk of a blood clot with some (not all) types of HRT. Taking some types of combined HRT may be associated with a higher risk of breast cancer (but the risk of breast cancer is higher for women who are obese or drink a moderate amount of alcohol). If you have a history of blood clots, liver disease or migraine, then there is a small risk of clotting if taking oestrogen in tablet form, but taking it in a patch, gel or spray is safe.

Are there any side effects?

There shouldn't be, but if there are they're relatively uncommon; they can include breast tenderness or bleeding. Usually, side effects occur in the first few months of taking HRT and usually go away as your body gets used to the hormones.

In my survey a couple of women spoke of their experience of using HRT. It was clear that it isn't a magic wand and it can take time to get the right dosage that works for you so that you experience a dramatic enough change.

I've had to up my dose twice this year. I feel like I'm on a really shit rollercoaster that could break at any time but that you can't get off. It's worse than the early baby years, as at least people are sympathetic as 'you've just had a baby'. No one gets this as most people think menopause is for women who are older than forty-something.

I definitely feel better, but it doesn't mean I don't have bad days too. There's the physical side but of course there's also the emotional one, like feeling less relevant and forgotten, and HRT won't take those feelings away.

Alternatives to HRT

Aside from looking after yourself in terms of exercise, healthy food and reducing alcohol consumption, there are lots of supplements out there although many of them are unproven. This is especially true of supplements that have been designed and marketed at the menopausal market (they're also more expensive). Vitamin D is important, there's some evidence that folic acid can help, some women have found sage to be beneficial and others swear by fish oils and probiotics. It's definitely worth doing some research before you spend lots of money on supplements.

So, like many things, it's good to be prepared for the menopause. It's unavoidable – just like other aspects of getting older. Remember that every woman goes through it and there's support out there. Also, it will get better. Don't be scared. It'll be okay. Honestly.

One quote from my survey sums up the benefits of facing up to the menopause instead of hiding away from symptoms and hoping they'll disappear:

The thing is, I have suppressed symptoms for ages and tried not to think about it, but since contacting my GP and booking an appointment I feel a sense of relief. It's the relief of knowing that I've nothing to hide. It's the relief of sharing it.

The more we share it, the less of a taboo it becomes and then hopefully our daughters' generation won't feel so fearful when they go through it and they'll get to the beach much more quickly.

Ten clues that you're actually getting on a bit

1. You have forgotten how to dance properly and so do a weird side-step and clap your hands just like your nan used to at weddings.
2. Your biggest pleasure is taking your bra off in the evening.
3. You walk into a room looking for something but then forget what you were looking for and walk back out.
4. You spend an inordinate amount of time looking for your glasses.
5. You scrutinise people's faces to try and work out what work they've had done.
6. You sigh a lot, and when you sit down you say out loud, 'There we go.'
7. You plan what you'll have for dinner whilst eating breakfast.
8. Your wee smells more intense somehow.
9. You fantasise about old boyfriends from the past and wonder what they're doing these days.
10. You sometimes have to turn 6Music down because when they play rave music it puts you in a strange time warp trance and you burn the fish fingers you're making for the kids' tea.

Where are the mid-life role models (who are NOT Helen Mirren)?

I sometimes feel like whenever the word 'older woman' pops up in the media then the self-same group of women gets rolled out. Oh, here's Helen Mirren. Here's Dame Judi Dench. Here's Jane Fonda. There is rarely any ethnic diversity (and this is a huge issue, as is the issue of privilege). And on top of that, many of the women are fabulous but not necessarily in the forty/fifty age bracket anymore. It's not enough to just cast one woman with long grey hair in a fashion spread and feel like you've ticked the box. Then the other thing is that many women in their forties and fifties who are in the public eye tend to brush over the ageing part. They might make some passing, lighthearted reference to the menopause and having hot flushes, but beyond that the language is always around how confident they feel, how carefree, how they can say what they want now they're older. I get that, but how about we also show some of the more challenging sides of ageing?

So, who are the aspirational role models for the forty- and fifty-something woman? These are mine.

Courtney Love

I know she's a controversial figure and she's had a very hedonistic lifestyle, but many forget that she is/was a rock frontwoman extraordinaire. The thing I like most about her is the fact that she doesn't care what people think and hasn't for some time now. She's not just saying it in an interview with *Red* magazine or to hawk some expensive face cream.

Kathy Burke

I've always admired Kathy Burke because she strikes me as the kind of woman who really doesn't give a crap about what others think of her. She speaks her mind, is an excellent actress and is the kind of woman you want to share tea and cake with whilst setting the world to rights. She has also been open about how horrendous her experience of the menopause was and admitted she hated being a woman during this time because she felt so isolated. Maybe Kathy has off days when she worries about how people perceive her, but I wish I could channel a small bit of her energy (in fact, that might be the title of my next book: 'How We Can Resolve Insecurity by Channelling More Kathy Burke').

Oprah

She is worth 2.6 billion dollars. She is one of the most powerful women in the entire world. She likes a book and the entire world reads the book. She is influential but not in a creepy way. She is funny and lighthearted and positive. She doesn't get grumpy – not that there's anything wrong with being grumpy, of course. She tackles important political issues. She has had the same best friend for years. The list of accolades goes on and on...

Sharon Horgan

I loved *Catastrophe*. And *Pulling*. I have tried to message her several times on Instagram, hoping that she'd reply and maybe read one of my blogs or books, but to no avail (she thinks I'm a stalker and she's right). I like her sense of style. I like the way she writes. I like the fact that she makes impending doom and disaster so funny. End of.

Kerry Washington

Did you watch *Little Fires Everywhere* and marvel at Kerry Washington's performance? I found that I couldn't tear my eyes away from her. She totally outshone everyone else and managed to be complex, flawed and totally relatable (with a realistic depiction of motherhood that doesn't shy away from being crap at times and making mistakes, which is nice as there is still not enough of this kind of motherhood depicted on screen). She aced it in *Scandal*, which I binge-watched in one go, and she's apparently the eighth highest-paid television actress, which in an industry that often pays women far less is no mean feat.

Kathryn Hahn

This actress played Raquel Fein in *Transparent*, and more recently played Dessa in *I Know This Much is True* with Mark Ruffalo. She was also in *I Love Dick* with Kevin Bacon. And *Bad Moms* (which was a bit shit, but I liked the premise of it). I don't actually know what her real-life persona is, but she always plays strong, ballsy women and I love her for it. She has a great fashion sense. I also love her in the film about a couple struggling with infertility called *Private Life*. I haven't actually seen any drama that shows an older woman who is struggling with having kids and isn't evil. The film is both funny and very honest in showing the bastard-ness of fertility treatment and how it saps the life out of you and your relationship.

Helena Bonham Carter

She dresses how she likes. She is a brilliant actress. For a long time I thought she held the secret to a successful long-term relationship because she lived in a separate house to her partner Tim Burton (but they sadly split up). I can't wear any of the clothing combinations she champions because I'd look mad, but she carries everything off with aplomb. I WISH SHE WAS MY FRIEND.

CHAPTER SEVEN

Anxiety, You Ain't My Pal

Me, Mindfulness and Meditation

As soon as I hit forty, my anxiety levels went through the roof. Much of it was related to having recently had a baby, going through fertility treatment and miscarriages, losing my status at work after having a fairly high-flying career, and ageing. I started to doubt everything. *I was a lousy mother. I was a massive underachiever. I wasn't clever enough. My body was a flop.* After having my second daughter, I felt quite good initially. People congratulated me on how well I was doing. I was on the school run, writing articles, I was even fitting in the odd run here and there. I had two books coming out. I had another child, which was exactly what I'd longed for. There was that little voice saying, '*You should be happy, mate. Smile. What have you got to complain about?*' Then suddenly, about six months in, I got anxiety on an epic scale. If I could draw a diagram with my keyboard that represented my feelings it would look something like this:

£@(>X£@&^%$£@!)(*&^%$

And I wanted to feel more like this:

Or perhaps even this:

!!!!!!!!!!!!!!!!!!!!!!!!!!!!!!!!!!!!

A typical day in the world of an anxious person

6am: Woken by crying baby after another sleepless night. Rush to toilet with upset tummy. Have to poo madly, which immediately makes me worry that I am dying/have stomach cancer/something is badly wrong with me.

6.30am: Crawl back into bed, heart beating wildly and on the verge of tears. Overwhelming feelings of fear, like someone is about to charge into the bedroom and hit me around the head with a baseball bat. Want to go back to sleep just to shut away these feelings again.

7am–9.30am: Try and get kids ready for school/playgroup, all the time fighting stomach palpitations and a sense of impending doom. Go to toilet again. Drink coffee, which makes everything much worse but is necessary because I'm feeling so tired with no energy to get through day.

9.30am–1pm: Go to baby group and try and make chit-chat about latest deals in Lidl ('Did you know they're selling inflatable canoes this week?') and baby-led weaning. Getting humming in ears and feel like I'm underwater. Why is everyone else acting normally when I'm dying from some stomach complaint and my baby is skinny and doesn't seem to be able to hold her head up yet? One mum bragging about how her kid can eat on his own at two months sends me right over the edge of the precipice. Have to visit toilet again.

1pm–6pm: The best part of the day – anxiety subsiding whilst baby naps and I get down to some writing and then go to the park and feel almost normal. Fearful feelings will return. Go through routine of school run, chatting to mums in the park, never really mentioning what's going on for fear people will think I'm losing my marbles. Stomach troubles return briefly.

6pm–10pm: Feelings of overwhelm return as get near to bedtime. Catastrophising about worst-case scenarios (i.e. *What if I'm an awful parent? What if I never work again? What if I feel like this in the morning? Why can't baby hold her head up? Why are they selling canoes, and do I need to purchase one? But when would I use it?*) and the whole thing starts again.

It took me a while to talk about how I was feeling. A friend recommended that I get some proper support rather than just soldier on. I was finding the symptoms debilitating. I had moments when I felt okay but they were few and far between. I'd hoped they'd go away but found as time went on, I got more anxious at the very prospect of getting anxious.

Thankfully, more people are talking about mental health, but nonetheless there is still a stigma attached to anxiety – it's certainly not something you want to talk about at work. Later I recognised that the anxiety had been embedded in my psyche for years. I'd sometimes managed to harness the fear and it helped me to do great presentations and get shit done but there'd been other times when I'd felt immobilised and my head wouldn't stop thinking and overthinking things that colleagues said or the sub-text of a certain email. Many women experience anxiety but on the outside look completely normal. Recently I was in the park with a woman who I'd observed to be successful (she was a TV producer), always impeccably dressed, organised (the kind of mum who has baked snacks in the oven and brought them in a nice, clean Tupperware). 'I have never felt so anxious in my life,' she said, as we watched our kids go down the slide. It just flopped out of her mouth. I realised that anxiety isn't always visible. In fact, a high-functioning person may fight their anxious feelings through trying to project a perfect vision of themselves and their lives to the outside world. I have friends who are anxious but their homes are immaculate (cleaning is sometimes a good outlet for anxiety if you feel your life is out of control). I know women who can present in front of an audience of twenty people but are catastrophising about what will go wrong in five minutes' time. After the birth of my second baby, I didn't show any visible signs of anxiety. For years previously I thought it was fairly normal that my hands sweated excessively or I couldn't breathe as I sat down to give a presentation. The problem is that the fight or flight response is activated whenever we feel under threat, and if we're about to do a big thing like a presentation, then it's normal to have heart palpitations and sweaty hands – in fact it's strange if you feel nothing at all. The difficulty is if you experience these kind of symptoms frequently and without any trigger. Then you can enter into a wormhole of negativity – feeling worried about the symptoms, the symptoms getting worse and then worrying about them some more.

Back to me with anxiety and a new baby... Not having any work structure, the only escape I had was getting out of the house. I would get up early, shower and be out by about 8.30. I was lucky in that I met another mum who I got on with (and who was also experiencing anxiety). Together we'd charge off to play groups and then lunch – both of us trying to avoid going home or stopping as we knew that would be when the obsessive thoughts would come raining down. It was frightening when I caught sight of my reflection, because I looked like somebody about to be fired out of a cannon and into the Milky Way.

My worries were linked to my daughter's feeding. She was headstrong and was constantly rejecting her bottle of milk.

'What if she starves?' I'd bleat to my partner. 'She's not had a bottle now for four hours.' My heart would be hammering in my chest and I could barely breathe.

'She'll be fine. She's not going to starve herself.'

'But what if she does? What if she never drinks milk again and then she'll have to go to hospital and have a tube and maybe pick up some awful bug. What if that happens?'

I found it exhausting to always be in a state of high panic. I found some solace in talking to other people, usually mums I met in the park. I'd suddenly blurt out my fears and then they'd come out with some other fears that they were carrying deep inside and immediately we connected and I felt less alone. Anxiety is especially common post-baby but it also crops up before and during menopause or at particular times of the month. The outside world plays a part – the Covid-19 pandemic has made people with anxiety feel like their worst fears have finally been realised. Much of the advice around anxiety is about trying to differentiate between things you can control and those you can't – right now, and for the past few months, everything has felt out of our control and there's no clear way forward, which makes things frightening and disorientating for everyone. My fear and anxiety are always present – it's like a sneering crocodile with its snout (do they have snouts?) poking out of the water. It hides for a few days but then it suddenly pops up, grabs me by the neck and takes me for a spin. It doesn't eat me though. It isn't powerful enough to do that.

I now have a conversation with my anxiety to try and create some distance.

> **Me:** *Oh, right, it's you again and you're going to give me a bad tummy, yeah?*
>
> **Anxiety:** *Yeah, I'm going to give you a really bad tummy and then I'm going to get your heart going off, and basically you're going to feel sick too.*
>
> **Me:** *Okay, I know those feelings. I'm going to carry on regardless because I have things to do today.*
>
> **Anxiety:** *I'm not happy with that. I want you to lie on the floor.*

Me: *I'm in Lidl and there's kayaks on special offer which I'm tempted to buy and I need to get some cat food.*

Anxiety: *But your kid looks like it's coming down with something.*

Me: [Looking at kid in buggy who looks fine as far as I can tell] *She's okay. Go and bother someone else, will you?*

Anxiety: *You'll drown if you get that kayak. You can't do water sports. You hate your legs, remember? You'll have to get a wetsuit and then you'll spend too much and you've not got any work on the horizon.*

Me: *You may be right, but I'm going to get a small coffee. Bye for now.*

Experiences of anxiety can get worse as we enter menopause. I know that there is no 'fixing it' and it's likely I'll have to learn to live with it. I spoke to Dr Becky Quicke, a psychotherapist who specialises in speaking to women who are in peri-menopause and menopause. She said:

Women go through three massive initiations: menarchy, when we start our periods and change from a child into a new hormonal identity; then the next initiation is motherhood and this signifies a death of a part of us and a birth of a new part of us – as mothers: next is peri-menopause and menopause and our hormones fluctuate and change significantly during these times. We forget that we're mammals and deeply motivated to maintain our species. So, at these three points – menarachy, motherhood and menopause – we are extremely precious to the survival of our species. Our hormones change to dial up a sense of threat, and in essence if we look at it another way, we're precious at peri-menopause.

One of the issues is that women aren't made to feel 'precious' at this phase of their lives. Instead, they're being flung lots of unhelpful messages about the way they look, what they should be doing with their lives, how they should behave, and ultimately how the future is going to net out. This can often spark off anxiety as we're comparing ourselves to the messages we're receiving from popular culture, from advertising, from friends, and feeling that we're not good enough, not productive, not achieving. We experience feelings of depression or pessimism about the future, a sense that the future doesn't hold as much interesting stuff anymore and we are essentially going to be overlooked and our life is finished.

Techniques to try...

We can learn useful lessons from whales

Anxiety can be linked to a sense that our life is washed up and finished, because this is how we are made to feel by society as a whole. Dr Quicke explains:

> Biologically and evolutionarily we are mammals, and the only other species in the animal kingdom where the females live beyond the menopause are whales.[1] Whales don't have the brain development that we have and haven't been through the same social conditioning. So female whales that go through menopause become the leaders of their pod. They lead their pod to the best place in the sea, at the right times of the year, so their pod can have the food they need. They have all that wisdom from the years they've been reproducing and learning about the seas.

---

1 The only species that live beyond their reproductive years that we know of are **humans**, **short-finned pilot whales**, and **killer whales**. In all three species, females lose the ability to have children but continue living for decades afterwards.

Whales don't get put on the scrap heap once they get past that initiation into menopause. Equally, they're not made to feel competitive with other whales in terms of how many barnacles they have on their chin or how big their whale kitchen extension is. THEY ARE CELEBRATED AND BECOME LEADERS. As we get into our forties and approach menopause (aside from the hormonal changes that are making us feel that way), we are made to feel like we have zero function – no longer attractive, no longer fertile, no longer capable of meaningful work – and so really we need to be more like whales. Dr Quicke elaborates:

> The thing is, we have an important role to maintain our species. A deep driver but it's shut off. And yes, we do see post-menopausal women who are setting up charities and leading their communities, their families, sharing their wisdom, but there's a process to get there. There's a shedding and a need to let go and transform.

What I've learnt from talking to different experts in this field is that there isn't one 'process' that gets you through but instead there are many tools. The first is acknowledging that you're going through a transformative time rather than pretending everything is as it was before. It's about finding emotional support from your family and friends and support groups. (You could sign up for the 'How to Be a Boss at Ageing' FB group, for example, and meet other women in a similar phase of life.) Then it's about working through past trauma and addressing it. This might be through seeing a qualified therapist and finally working through stuff that you've shoved under the carpet to fester for years. It's also about using practical tools like mindfulness and meditation and yoga and good sleep and supplements. All these things will help you feel better and build you back up again.

We need to be more in tune with our bodies

I've included a few tools at the end of this chapter that can help ease anxiety. One thing I've discovered is the importance of being more aware of what's going on in my body and brain rather than trying to run away from my feelings (by scrolling Instagram, online shopping, buying kayaks in Lidl). One of the benefits of getting older is that I can more readily see patterns in my behaviour. So, I find that mornings are particularly bad for me – oh, and last thing at night too. So, on a typical morning, I might wake up and immediately feel a sense of fear around the day ahead. Usually this is shaped by the fact that my partner leaves for work super early and I have both girls on my own, need to get them ready for school/childcare and then get on with work (and at this particular time, the work is stressful and I'm telling myself I can't do it because it's too hard). So, my brain is pinging all these messages at me about not being able to cope, how the day is going to be too hard for me to manage, how things are going to go wrong – and this is usually before I've even set foot outside the bedroom. It's exacerbated by the fact that my kids are young and so I don't wake up gradually but instead hear one of them screaming (which immediately gets those fight or flight responses kicked into action).

Before I realised this scenario was a trigger, I just let the feelings take over. I'd run around like mad – almost believing that the more quickly I moved and stayed on top of things, the more likely I'd be able to 'out-run' the fact that my stomach was churning and my heart was thundering in my chest. Now, most mornings I try to wake a tiny bit earlier so I can listen to a short meditation on my phone before the kids start yelling. If they do wake me up, then I try to slow myself down a bit. I tell myself some kind things – things that a friend would say to me: *You're doing great. Everything is fine. One step at a time* – that kind of thing. If the anxiety is particularly bad, I take the kids downstairs, put the TV on (to be honest the TV goes on whatever my state of mind is, because they wake up so, so early) and then lie on the sofa and listen to a quick meditation (I love the Clementine app because it has short meditations on there). I think about the things that will make me feel better rather than focusing on thoughts that make me feel worse. I have a coffee but I don't have more than two. I have a walk get some fresh air. If I'm sat at my laptop and feeling crap, I get up, go into the garden and try and focus on a few specific things. These are tools that I've learnt over time. Everyone will be different in terms of what works for them, but I know that speeding up my pace, worrying about my symptoms, catastrophising about the day… all these things will increase my anxious feelings. One big revelation for me was the fact that anxiety is entirely normal. Everyone has it to some degree or other. And importantly, it's not something you'll ever really get shot of. This may sound depressing, but for me it just makes me more committed to not letting it stop me from doing the things I have to do each day.

NB: It's worth noting that if your anxiety is crippling and you can't do the things that you have to do each day, then that's not your fault and you need to seek out expert help. Speak to your GP. The anxiety I experience is one that I can handle most of the time on my own. I've had to seek help before though, and through counselling I started to assemble my own tool kit. I wouldn't feel ashamed if the need arose to seek help again. I know that mental health issues are important – I come from a background where I lost my step-mum and half-sister to suicide, so perhaps I'm more likely to seek professional help than others. I sincerely believe that they would both be alive today if my step-mum had had more professional support at the time. This makes my heart break to be honest.

As women enter their mid-forties, we're often just as busy and overwhelmed as we were in our thirties. Motherhood might have come later, we're trying to forge ahead with our careers, relationships may be breaking down, and this means by the time we enter the peri-menopause we're totally burnt out and knackered. It pays to become more familiar with our cycles and what's going on in our bodies so we can plan things accordingly. We can't always do this, but sometimes just knowing that hormonally we are likely to feel a certain way (and it's not just coming from nowhere) can help us navigate through the feelings and anxiety.

Dr Quicke sees this in the women that come to see her for help and has also experienced it herself:

> Many of us are coming to peri-menopause with a depleted adrenal system, and I had this myself. I was burnt out and then I got more aware of my cycle. And the thing is, we don't need to stop completely at certain times of the month but we need to be savvy as to when we do things. There are phases in the cycle where we are primed to be out there and doing all the things, and there are phases where we are not. In my experience – and it's the experience of many – our menstrual cycles become heightened and we need to rest during menstruation because then we're able to do the things when we're ovulating. We need to tune into our bodies more.

Recognise that past trauma and the impact it has on our mental health

Our forties and fifties are often the time when we can't keep going at the same pace and the hormones can bring the crows home to roost. Again, this can create anxiety that is manifesting from things that have happened earlier in our lives. Dr Quicke expands on this:

> We've typically been go, go, go and fixated on doing everything in our twenties and thirties. We get to this phase in our forties and we're exhausted keeping it all boxed off. Our hormones crack

us open and this stuff rises to the top. We can't keep the trauma quiet. Or it might be that the body experiencing these changes associates it with a difficult time in our lives – it remembers how it feels to be all over the place and the feelings rise up again. It can be because we've pushed it away and then it comes back.

For me personally, I know my anxiety is shaped by things that happened when I was in my teens – losing my step-mum and sister, then more recently losing my dad unexpectedly. All these things are related. I know that I possibly need to talk to a therapist about what happened in my teens and how I never faced up to the trauma in my family. I escaped instead into a world of hedonism. Then I buried myself in work. Then came the desire to get pregnant and endless fertility treatment. Then BOOM –I was in my forties and the trauma returned, exacerbated by the fact that my father was the only one who understood what had happened and was no longer around. I was ready to talk about it, but he'd gone. I know that this won't just go away and I probably need to talk to someone about it. I'm also fearful about bringing the whole thing out into the open. The thing is, trauma doesn't disappear and it'll rear its head somewhere along the line. Speaking to a specialist can really help.

Don't give up (like Thom Yorke does in that video)

Do you remember right at the beginning of the book when I talked about the Radiohead video where Thom Yorke lies face down on the pavement? We've all had days when life overwhelms us, and this, combined with fluctuating hormones, dealing with society, dealing with baggage, dealing with mountains of admin (and remembering the password for the Wifi which was written down somewhere but has been ripped up and chucked in the bin)… Well, there's certainly a sense on bad days that it would be easier to GIVE UP. And sometimes this is required. Dr Quicke feels we need to give in to these feelings at times instead of trying to brush them under the carpet: 'The lying on the floor and surrendering is normal. We have these tricky brains that want to judge, and it's not always helpful.' She also firmly believes that it's about living with difficult feelings rather than trying to get rid of them completely, which is unrealistic:

> Society has demonised anxiety and it's about trying to get rid of it. So, we say to ourselves that we shouldn't be feeling like this and we need to 'master it' and 'fight anxiety', and that's one of the biggest issues we face because we become anxious because we feel anxious. The more we try and get rid of anxiety, the stronger it becomes. What you resist persists.

So, yes, it's fine some days to take stock and acknowledge that you're having a bad time. It's also good to have tools that can help you get up off the floor and move towards the things you want in life. Dr Quicke continues:

> So the new way of understanding human-ness is that we all experience anxiety but to what extent does it get in the way of moving towards what you want to do? It may be that sometimes you are experiencing anxiety and it's needed and there are other times when it's holding you back.

Try grounding techniques when things are tough

There are times when the physical symptoms – the heart palpitations, the panic, the bad tummy, the sense of doom – can be overwhelming. Dr Quicke's advice is to bring yourself into the present:

> In that moment you need to regulate the body. One of the key skills is to ground yourself in the present. That's where mindfulness

comes in. Our mind is overwhelmed. It's about becoming more grounded. It's useful to open up your senses, and I quite often say to people to focus on the sensation of your feet being on the ground or a certain touch or smell. Smell is a great one, actually. It helps us regulate ourselves. So, an example would be if your child is having a massive tantrum and you can feel yourself getting worked up, then have a handwash that you love the smell of and wash your hands. It brings the body down a bit and grounds you in your senses again.

Another technique which has served me well in the past is trying to spot three things in my line of vision and to name these things. So, for instance, you could say to yourself: *bird, tree, sky*. Then try and listen for three sounds and name these too, so: *car driving past, wind in the trees, child talking*. Finally, try and feel three things with your senses, so: *cold on my face, texture of my jacket between my fingers, and soles of my shoes on the pavement*. Just doing this exercise brings you back into your body and stops you in your tracks. If you see me muttering under my breath, then it's likely that this is what I'm doing. I recently tried it out in Tesco when I was having a particularly bad time, and it worked. I also find that it gives me something practical to do when I'm feeling out of control. The panic then tends to gradually subside.

HRT can work well for some women in highly anxious states

You need to work out whether HRT is right for you personally, but anxiety is often related to hormonal changes, so rebalancing these can help, especially if the anxiety levels are high. Dr Quicke explains how HRT can be helpful if anxiety levels are high:

> Anxiety in peri-menopause and menopause is different because of the hormonal aspect. If women are interested and able [to take

it], HRT can be a helpful way to dial this anxiety down. GPs talk about using HRT initially, then moving onto examination, transformation and other techniques and looking at how we respond to sensations when we're having difficult feelings.' To try and problem-solve is not helpful. It keeps us trapped. It's about learning and being flexible so you can respond to the thoughts and sensations in a flexible way that means it doesn't hold us back.

In essence, we need to change our relationship with anxiety. It's not something that magically disappears but there are things we can do to help ourselves. We can think like the whales: coming into our own, leading our communities, leading our families, feeling like we have all the knowledge and the know-how; but if this makes you feel pressured and more anxious, then just think of yourself as a peaceful, mindful whale, swimming in the ocean, with the waves passing over your silky skin as your tail fin delicately breaks the surface and you then go back down to the sea bed for a twenty-minute lie-down.

Some things that have helped me when things have got tough anxiety-wise

Counselling

I hesitated to get in touch with the NHS because I didn't think my anxiety was severe enough. But then I realised that it was severe enough for me to be anxious about it and thankfully I was lucky enough to get CBT sessions through the NHS. These helped. I was given practical tools I could use when I was feeling wobbly. I haven't always kept going with these tools because I'm lazy but I know that if my anxiety returns, I can use them again. You can contact your GP and get more information on this. There can be a long waiting list, but I was prioritised because I was a new mum. You can obviously go private too. (For more details, look at www.bacp.co.uk, the website for the British Association for Counselling and Psychotherapy.)

Meditation

My step-mum and dad meditated when I was growing up, and because I liked to reject most of the things they did, I avoided meditation until I got into my forties. Now I'm not into long sessions but if I'm feeling a bit crap and on edge, I'll take five or ten minutes and just sit. There are lots of apps that I've found helpful in bringing short meditation sessions into my everyday routine. If I'm having a particularly bad day, then I'll listen to a meditation on headphones as I return from the school run. I use apps like Clementine, Headspace, Buddifhy and Calm. Part of the reason I never used to meditate was because I didn't feel I had enough time. A lot of people advise you do it first thing in the morning, but since my kids wake at 5.30am and setting an alarm before that time feels unnatural, I have a couple of apps I can use if I get a spare five or ten minutes once the kids are in bed or if I'm travelling or can just sit in the toilet for a couple of minutes. Part of it for me is just putting some distance between the things that I'm thinking and the way that I'm feeling. Sometimes just a reminder – for example, saying 'I am not my thoughts' – helps. I use that phrase a lot. As well as 'FOR FUCK'S SAKE' and 'CAN YOU PLEASE BRUSH YOUR TEETH OR THERE WILL BE NO SCREEN TIME TODAY'.

Mindfulness

Mindfulness is the practice of paying attention to your thoughts but not allowing yourself to get caught up and carried away. It's as if you're a third person and you're just observing the positive and negative thoughts that pop into your brain, and letting them float past. It's about getting immersed in the moment. So if you're having a shower, it's about just feeling the water on your body and the scent of the shower gel, and not thinking about whether you need to purchase a canoe from Lidl or whether your boss is going to point out everything you've done wrong yet again. Ruby Wax has written a great book about mindfulness (see the Resources section). I still find being mindful challenging, but repeating some of my thought patterns out loud helps me create a bit of distance.

Exercise is your friend

If you're one of those people that spends too much time in your head – too much time ruminating – then exercise is an effective way to calm down and get into your body again. It also gives you a natural rush of endorphins. I'm hopeless at yoga as I have zero flexibility and a hunched back from years sitting at a computer, but still, yoga has helped. Yoga with Adrienne is a great app and she has an extensive playlist on YouTube, including yoga practices for anxiety. They're often only fifteen minutes, so can be done first thing or last thing at night. Running has been helpful, and also doing thirty-minute workouts (I have put a link to the classes I do at the back of the book). Basically, you think that you aren't capable of exercising because you feel so anxious, but it's actually quite hard to run and feel those emotions at the same time (unless you're being chased by a bear, but that's not very likely in West London).

Breathing

Sometimes just lying on the floor and making sure you're breathing properly is the most helpful thing. There are loads of resources on how to use breath more effectively when you're feeling overwhelmed. We tend to breathe fast and shallow when we're anxious, so practising techniques like the 4-5-7 breath can really help. Breathe in for four counts, hold for five counts and exhale for seven. Do this about four times with your eyes shut and you should feel much calmer (it was developed by Dr Andrew Weill and there are lots of videos of him talking it through).

Podcasts

I'm a massive Adam Buxton fan and his podcast (The Adam Buxton Podcast), which is probably the most established one I know, helped me get through my post-baby anxiety. There were days when reading about anxiety and then doing exercises to help anxiety were just making me feel more anxious. Listening to this podcast was an escape – the silly jingles and lunatic songs and the interviews, which are always very light and funny but also have lots of poignant moments. I don't feel like I'm being massively original here but one thing I will say is that finding content that isn't always about mental health can be helpful (or it was for me as I started to get overly obsessed in many ways). I like to listen to interviews as this helps me gain perspective and take a step away from being inside my own head.

There are more podcasts in the Resources section of this book.

Anxiety may always be with you, but you can learn to live with it and navigate your way through. It will come and go. It's just a case of seeking help if it gets out of control and learning more about the tools that will help you long term.

What's the deal with mysticism?
Can it be helpful to me?

Let me be clear here and say that I'm not an expert in this area and I can't read Tarot cards and I don't have many rituals aside from the following:

- I have a green, marble Buddha which I rub each time I walk past. I rubbed it whilst I was going through IVF and on the night that my dad died I rubbed it multiple times. So the Buddha may have helped with fertility but didn't stop me losing dad. I now feel less confident that he's manifesting real change in my life.
- I always touch the side of my head if I see a magpie.
- I won't walk under ladders and will cross the road if I see a black cat coming towards me.
- I sleep with my dad's old hankie under my pillow and am obsessive about not losing this.

The above are not really rituals as such. They are just small behaviours that make me feel more in control and connect me to something bigger (aside from the hankie under the pillow, which is more about grief and the comfort I get from having something that belonged to my dad close by).

The thing is, rituals, superstitions and magic are useful if you think they are. That is to say, if they make you feel better and if they don't harm anyone else. So, eating live bats isn't a good ritual but writing a negative thought that your inner critic keeps saying on a piece of paper and then burning that paper is a good ritual (if it makes you feel better). If you think about life as being hectic and anxiety-making, then following moon cycles and rituals might help ground you. They may help you remember that there are bigger forces out there, even if we don't know what they are exactly or maybe don't always believe in them but sometimes do.

When I was in my early thirties, visiting Glastonbury (the town, not the festival), I was fascinated but also semi-appalled by the shops selling expensive crystals, sage-burning contraptions, and books about witches and spells. It was an entire industry I'd been unaware of. I noticed there was a certain kind of woman (usually post-forty) who frequented these shops: the type that wore long, black, tassled skirts, had dark, smudged eyeliner and ponged of patchouli oil and herbal cigarettes and who possibly listened to bands like Steeleye Span (Google them – they're actually quite good, but my dad played them a bit and maybe put me off when I was a child) and olde worlde English folk music (i.e. songs about tragic young girls who got lost on the clifftops and fell into ditches playing the fiddle).

I dismissed all of it as hokum because I was a capitalist pig and worked in market research and liked The Slug & Lettuce too much. Now I'm older and like burning candles (but can't afford Diptique ones anymore so have to make do with Tesco ones shoved into a used Diptique candle holder) and the odd ritual here and there, it's all coming back onto my radar. The thing is, people have always been suspicious of women who are interested in mysticism (and many women were of course killed if they were thought to be witches). As we all desperately root around for some kind of meaning as we get older and perhaps find it hard to believe in God but want to feel some sort of spiritual connection, well that's where mysticism comes in. I'm aware that I'm giving a very superficial description of what it's all about, but there are of course dozens of books dedicated to the subject. I spoke to Emma

Howarth (@mysticalthinking on Instagram), who gave me a bit more background.

>**Anniki:** So, Emma, why do you think women are becoming more interested in mysticism and moon cycles and the solstice and rituals? Is it because of a lack of authority figures and the decline of religion?
>
>**Emma:** I think that's a big part of it, YES. And because life is so hectic and busy... sometimes it's nice to tap into that ancient wisdom and connect with something bigger... but without all the God stuff. It's all about connecting with nature and finding a sense of peace and making sense of the world! Also learning to trust ourselves and our own intuition too.
>
>**Anniki:** What do you think are the benefits of opening up this side of your life?
>
>**Emma:** It has helped me to chill out A LOT... I find it easier to just let something go now... and just know it wasn't meant for me. Less comparison to other people and thinking they are doing better than me, and more time to notice the small stuff. It's also fun! We're all trying to drink less and live healthier lives... but guided meditations and sound baths and ceremonies and rituals can be just as diverting as a bottle of rosé. I really like the 'something to do' that isn't just a going-to-a-bar-element.
>
>**Anniki:** Thinking about rituals, what kind of accessible things can women do to experiment with mysticism?
>
>**Emma:** I'd start with learning about the moon – it's such an interesting way to live in tune with nature and come to understand that everything happens in cycles. We're not designed to be ON IT all the time. Living by the moon is like a natural reminder of that which is helpful. Basically, the waxing phase is for getting stuff done; the full moon is magic manifestation and letting go; then the waning phase is

all about retreating, letting go, learning, gathering strength; and the new moon is intention setting and starting again. I think of it as a mini monthly New Year! Way better than just getting the one chance to up your game each year.

Anniki: Finally, does this stuff work? Do you feel it helps to improve our lives and make us feel more in control during difficult times?

Emma: Absolutely YES. Discovering and rediscovering this stuff has changed my life for the better. It's also made me feel a bit like I can get what I want just by believing in it… which is pleasing!

A tribute to self-help – from a lifelong fan

I eat self-help books up like a greedy pig with its head in a bucket of slop. I've been doing so since a young age. The first one I read was *Feel the Fear and Do it Anyway* by Susan Jeffers. I was addicted to that one because I felt like every day I was letting fear dominate my life. On bad days I was too frightened to even go to the supermarket. I was living in Amsterdam with my boyfriend, who'd been in a famous Goth band and was now making dance music. I had a job cleaning a music studio in the centre of town and was clubbing about four times a week. I watched a lot of TV – mainly old-school Oprah where she had massive hair and big shoulder-padded skirt suits. I was stuck in a rut, recovering from trauma that I'd been through in my teens, and my life felt bleak (when I wasn't going out and off my nuts that is). I underlined key phrases in the book and then tried to implement them. I wasn't very good at this, but some of the theory stuck with me. The key gist of the book is that you are always going to feel afraid of change, and if you wait for the fear to disappear, then you'll never do anything. So, the thing is, you have to acknowledge the fear and just go ahead and do it anyway. This was a big piece of learning for me because I thought everyone around me wasn't afraid and was doing things because they were more confident than I was. What I hadn't realised was that, to a greater or lesser extent, everyone is afraid – it's just the extent to which they let that fear get in the way of what they want to achieve. I still apply this to my life now. If I'm talking at an event or doing a podcast interview, I accept that the butterflies in my stomach and rapid heartbeat are completely normal and aren't going to go away until about halfway through whatever I'm doing. Sometimes my hands will shake and sometimes I'll get breathless. Now I am familiar with these things and just get on with it anyway.

Back in those teenage years in Amsterdam, once I'd really had enough of doing drugs/no routine/eating too many chips with mayonnaise/watching too much Oprah, I also took action (i.e. eventually returning to the UK and sitting my A levels in one year and then getting a job). I was scared and worried that I was making the wrong decision but I'd also absorbed some of those messages from Susan Jeffers' book. There were other contributing factors too – the fact that I was depressed and bored and was living the life of a member of Guns N' Roses that wasn't sustainable, but even now I find the messages useful. Don't wait too long. Act. And acknowledge that you'll feel wobbly during this change.

This is still a good thing to say to yourself today (unless it's something dangerous, in which case there's a reason your body is telling you NOT to do it – and your body is RIGHT, so give it the respect it deserves and listen to it).

I always feel like the moment I buy a nice, fresh self-help book, my life is about to go off on a happier, more productive trajectory.

One of my favourite books was *The Secret*, which many people read and raved about when it first came out. I'm not going to rubbish the idea of manifestation but I can say that I did every single exercise in the book and my life didn't improve one jot. I kept ruminating about why this was – perhaps I was doing the manifesting wrong (another thing to feel anxious about). Perhaps my vibrations weren't intense enough. Since reading it, I've read many accounts of celebrities who wrote their wish to be megastars on slips of paper and hid them in shoeboxes or under their pillows. Jim Carrey wrote himself a cheque for a huge amount of money before he had any and then became a household name. (I tried this, too, after reading about it in a book all about manifesting money but I have yet to receive this amount – I'M PUTTING THIS OUT THERE, UNIVERSE, OKAY?)

The thing is, my dad was always down-to-earth and rational and had studied stoicism and philosophy, so there is definitely one side of myself that is cynical about manifestation. The other thing is, we only hear about the people who MANIFESTED STUFF AND IT CAME TRUE. We don't hear about Anniki Sommerville, working in market research, doing endless focus groups, dealing with infertility, migraine headaches and each night writing on a slip of paper things like 'I AM MARRIED TO DAVE GROHL AND LIVE IN THE HOLLYWOOD HILLS WITH SIX CHILDREN' (I didn't write that kind of stuff down… oh, hang on, I did). Or 'I AM MARIAN KEYES AND AM MARRIED TO DAVE GROHL AND LIVE IN THE HOLLYWOOD HILLS WITH SIX CHILDREN.' I'm not going to put manifesting to bed, because if it makes you feel better, then do it. It doesn't harm anyone. It only harms you if you truly believe that writing your wishes down on a piece of paper and putting them under your pillow is something you do instead of working at making your dreams a reality. You have to be lucky, yes. If you want to marry Dave Grohl, then you need luck and the right geographical location and to not be living in a suburb of West London where the house prices are reasonable because the local area mainly comprises kebab shops. You probably need to have some sort of role in the music industry rather than working on a new packaging proposition for a toilet roll and talking to groups of 40-something women about whether they want a puppy on the roll or a koala or a bear (this is what I spent about five years of my life doing – no joke).

I also tried the 'Gratitude Diary' and recently found one of these from when I was in my late thirties. I'd been frantically scraping the barrel most days to try and conjure up one positive thing to feel grateful for.

A typical entry looks something like this:

> I am grateful for the margarine on my toast this morning.
> I am grateful that I have a knife to put my margarine on my toast.
> I am grateful that I found a hairband to tie my hair back, because my neck was getting sweaty.
> I am grateful for the toilet paper that wiped my butt.

I was clutching at straws because I was undergoing fertility treatment and dealing with twice-a-day blood tests and unpleasant transvaginal ultrasounds (I always think that's the name of a 90's trance act) and I was feeling like my life was going nowhere.

I will say, however, that there are times when the gratitude exercise can really help. It's been *proven* to help, in fact. Here's a recent example of where it worked so you can see what it could potentially do for you. Back in October 2020, I was working in a job that wasn't quite working out for me. The reality of losing my dad was settling in and I was having a lot of negative thoughts around my writing and whether I'd ever actually get anywhere. And so I was basically caught in a negative whirlwind of crap – one negative thought cascading into the next negative one. I started trying to think about one thing at the end of each day that I'd enjoyed and found positive. I started with one thing because I knew it would be a challenge to find a lot of things. So I would lie in bed and think about the entire day in my head. Instead of pulling out the crap things – sending the wrong email to someone, getting a critical message from a colleague, forgetting it was 'World Green Hair Day' at school, I focused on something that had given me a lift, had made my heart sing a little. And the thing is, I always found something (and it was easier than coming up with a whole list, because sometimes life is tough and then it can feel like the 'clutching at straws' thing). So, I'd write something like 'The best moment today was when I picked up my youngest from the childminder and she ran out and hugged me and I sniffed the top of her head and gave her a massive hug.' And just this one positive observation helped me reframe the day. It also helped me remind myself what was important. So yes, it was annoying that I was getting a heap of shit at work from a colleague and the work wasn't ultimately what I wanted to do, but I had my kids and I loved them to death and they were the most important thing today, in this moment.

I've found that practising some sort of gratitude ultimately helps reframe your life – even if you can only list one thing that's positive, even if you struggle at first. The fact is that the more you practise it, the easier it becomes. It even translates to your posture when you walk down the street. I used to always have my eyes aimed at the pavement and I'd notice all the dog shit and the fact that someone had left a used condom on the ground (yes really) but now I try and notice the sky more or at least keep my gaze at eye-level for some of the time.

Many of the self-help books I've read have been helpful so I've listed a few in the Resources section later on. The one thing I've learnt is that you can shape your mindset, and self-help books have helped me learn that I can change my feelings if I am conscious of what's whirling around inside my brain.

How my attitudes to cleaning and housework have evolved with age

When I was younger, say in my early thirties, I was more paranoid about what people thought of the state of my home, and as a consequence I rarely invited anyone over. I was also guilty of picking things for my flat which I'd seen in home interiors magazines and thought were trendy but didn't actually like. I wanted my home to be immaculately clean and stylish. And if it wasn't going to be those two things, then I'd rather not have any visitors, thanks.

Now I'm older I care much less about what people think of my home. Whilst it sometimes depresses me when I get down on the floor to retrieve a toddler's shoe from under the sofa and notice there's a half-eaten orange under there that's completely dried up and is stuck to the floorboard, I don't feel mortified at the idea that a visitor might see it and what that might suggest about me as a woman/how successful I am/whether I'm stylish enough to be friends with them.

I have come to the firm conclusion that life is too short to clean my house all the time. I know there are people who disagree and think cleaning is great, but it never actually stops – this is especially true when you have young children. There is always mess to attend to. If you're a writer and you're working at home, then you essentially have a choice: a shiny kitchen floor or a chapter of a book written. I will always choose writing over cleaning. I don't believe anyone gets to the end of their life and declares, 'God I really wish my oven had been cleaner,' and then pops their clogs. I am what Kate Moss would no doubt call a BASIC BITCH when it comes to cleaning. Every Friday morning, I get out two cleaning products and I look at the clock. I then give myself roughly half an hour to clean the house. How do I do this? 'I have very poor standards' is the answer. I prioritise the kitchen and bathroom. And if I don't see it, then it doesn't exist to me. So I wipe things that are visible but would never bother to move furniture out of the way or investigate under beds unless I find myself under there looking for something –then I might bother to clean, but even then I will usually give up after ten minutes because it's so boring.

So, what does my cleaning and levels of cleaning say about my relationships? Here's a rough guide so you know roughly where you sit on the spectrum in terms of whether I care what you think about me or not…

- **I like you but don't know what kind of home you keep or how you'll judge me:** I'll clean the downstairs loo properly, including the floor. I will also dust everything within eyeshot and potentially run to the Londis to get cake (it will be Mr Kipling).
- **You're my mum/sister:** I won't bother doing anything at all but may replace the hand towel in the loo and pour some Ecover toilet cleaner in there (on a bad day it will be Toilet Duck as it's cheaper).
- **I think you're cool and want to get to know you more:** I'll clean the house from top to bottom just in case you ask for a tour. I will spend twenty minutes considering what book to leave out on my bedside table and will light at least one expensive candle (and will let it burn for the entirety of your visit but will be stressed at how fast it's going down and will extinguish it the moment you walk out the door). I will go to the baker or even try and make banana bread. I will sniff the hummus and consider serving it to you with some stale Tortilla chips. I will consider sorting out the kitchen cupboards in case you open anything, but then despair and just make sure you don't open anything – I serve you the entire time you're here.
- **We're old friends/I know you very well:** I will put toilet cleaner down the loo and make sure nobody has pooped

in there or left skid marks. I will give you a Maryland cookie that has seen better days (if you're going through a bad time, I will dash to the baker and spend some dosh and may even get you a pot plant if I have enough time).

- **I don't like you**: I won't let you into my home. We can talk on the doorstep or I will pretend I'm not in (this is only if I *really* don't like you, which is very rare, and you must be awful as I like most people).

CHAPTER EIGHT

Hedonism and Middle Age

Why Hangovers Are Hell as You Age

Let's be honest. Drinking when you're older is a nightmare…

Since I got past forty-five, I've noticed hangovers don't just last a day. Instead they go on for maybe three days, maybe even a week. The symptoms and fallout are becoming more complex, more… Well, awful, really.

Day one
- Wake up (get woken up by small child) at 5am.
- Feel suicidal with post-booze fear, pain and dread.
- Have feelings of remorse and anxiety which last entire day.
- Objective is to get through this first day with minimum amount of pain, so TV often involved for children, or any games which involve lying down (i.e. hospitals/beauty spa).

Day two
- Headache has subsided but entire body hurts and am haunted by underlying feeling that:
  ○ I have done something wrong.
  ○ I will be dying soon.
  ○ I am an awful parent.

- ○ I am ugly and fat.
- ○ Nobody likes me.
- ○ I have said something to someone that they have taken the wrong way and that's why they haven't put a kissing emoji on the last text they sent me.

Day three

- Cry for no reason when sad advert comes on the TV.
- Snap at kids when they are making the kind of noise kids make all the time.
- Feel entirely overwhelmed by mess and disorder in house and then get caught in more negative self-talk:
  - ○ I have done something wrong.
  - ○ I will be dying soon.
  - ○ I am an awful parent.
  - ○ I am ugly and fat.
  - ○ Nobody likes me.
  - ○ I have said something to someone that they have taken the wrong way and that's why they haven't put a kissing emoji on the last text they sent me.

And, yes, the reality is that as we get older, our bodies find it harder to deal with the fallout of booze. There's a reason why Shaun Ryder and Bez from the Happy Mondays now stay in and watch TV, as stars of *Celebrity Gogglebox* rather than taking massive amounts of ecstasy and smashing up dressing rooms. I have heard rumours that Kate Moss no longer drinks anymore – and wasn't she the iconic party animal for our generation? The thing is, there comes a time when every hedonist has to hang up those glitter-encrusted shoes and slip their feet into some Marks & Spencer's 'Comfy-Technology' slippers and start talking about the joys of turmeric lattes. I am now more likely to be found in a hot bath, listening to a podcast, than queuing at a bar with thundering music in the background (scratch that – I am more likely to be asleep as I go to bed at 10pm nowadays).

There is also something frowned upon when you're in your late forties and pissed. I am totally up for everyone doing what they want as long as it doesn't hurt anyone, but the older I've got the more I've realised that being drunk isn't a good look for me. It seems to make me more weepy, more argumentative, more depressed, and I don't get any of the giggly, silly, fun stuff. I start looking for old boyfriends online and then wonder why they've lost all their hair and then remember that I'm actually the same age and that we are all ageing and, oh no, we are going to have hangovers and we are going to die and it's the end of the world – put simply, drinking a lot doesn't make me happy.

And then there's the science around drinking and ageing. According to the Drinkwise website, as we age, muscle mass is replaced by fat tissue, which means that when you're older, drinking the same amount of booze as someone younger results in you having a higher blood alcohol concentration. You also process alcohol more slowly and it stays in your liver for longer, increasing the risk of damage. There is also an increased risk of accidents – putting you at higher risks of falls, slips or car crashes. Latest research has revealed that scientists have discovered that women produce smaller quantities than men of an enzyme called alcohol dehydrogenase (ADH) which is released in the liver and breaks down alcohol in the body. Women are also more likely to have higher levels of body fat, and lower amounts of body water, which means they have a more dramatic physiological response to drinking alcohol. So, put simply, we feel the effects of drinking more readily. And we are less efficient in breaking it down. There doesn't seem to be a huge amount of research into the effects of alcohol on women – and why is this? Is it because the alcohol industry is worth so much money and nobody wants to discover that drinking is far more harmful to women in the long term? It's a downer, yes, but it doesn't mean you have to give up entirely; but using booze as your main release/escape from life isn't a healthy long-term solution.

My relationship with alcohol has been troubled. I've found that because of the fallout and the three-day hangovers, there really is little point in doing it anymore. My father was an alcoholic and so I am very conscious that we may share some of the same genetic make-up (and I know I readily become addicted to things like buying embroidered tops on the Zara website and reading the sidebar of shame on the *Daily Mail*, even though it makes me feel dreadful).

Also, I've noticed that my evenings with drink are pretty much exactly the same as without drink.

Evening with drink
Watch TV with partner saying little and eating crisps.
Evening without drink
Watch TV with partner saying little and eating crisps.

Of course, there are the rare big nights out, but even then, the drinking is underwhelming. There is no longer anything REALLY craaazzzzy happening. Nobody is going off to the tattoo shop to get their belly buttons pierced. Nobody is snogging someone under the table. Nobody is having a big row with their best friend. The conversations get louder but are essentially about the same things: loft conversions, kitchen extensions, builder recommendations, teachers and teaching, house prices, good local restaurants and random news events depending on whatever is happening at that particular time. When I was in my twenties it wasn't unusual to go out of an evening and have a stranger come up and bite your arm (this happened to me), or your boob to pop out of your top as you were trying to get your wig out of a wind-machine. It wasn't all this dull old adult balls.

So, what's the point in drinking now? The problem is, the alternative is pretty joyless. You can talk about how nice it is to have fizzy water with a dash of lime in it or how Sipsmith is really cool (but basically you're paying booze prices for lemon squash). Isn't it depressing to just be sober all the time?

Actually, it's not that bad. I've had long periods of time, mainly due to trying to get pregnant, when I've stopped drinking. I also stopped when my daughters were little. I couldn't cope with no sleep and the fallout from alcohol. I am still flirting with sobriety as I felt so much better physically when I wasn't drinking.

Wine o'clock and resisting peer pressure

It's funny once you put your antennae up, you notice how much seductive messaging there is around women and booze. Especially mums and booze. When my daughter was a year old I noticed that all the mums around me were drinking more booze than I'd drunk back in university (an exaggeration, but they were certainly putting it away). At any barbecue or lunch, the mums were necking huge amounts of prosecco as if there was no tomorrow. The drinking would be compressed into a limited time frame (usually three to four hours) and then everyone would leave, swaying and trying to sober up as the reality of having to walk home, do the bedtime routine, etc. set in.

There's been a huge sobriety movement and lots of great books written about the positives of being sober (e.g. *The Joy of Being Sober* by Catherine Gray, *The Sober Diaries* by Clare Pooley, *From Rock Bottom to Sober Forever* by Susan Laurie). It's no longer seen as being uncool to not drink – if anything, there's a trend towards giving up. However, you may still be interrogated initially and come up against lots of defensiveness and comments like 'Well, I don't need to give up because I don't have a problem with booze and can stop whenever I like.' So, for me personally, as I've got past my mid-forties I've realised that there is a middle way. I have tried being 100 per cent sober, and whilst I felt fabulous physically, I still missed having a drink now and then, so I now only really drink once a week and try to keep it to one or two glasses of wine. I'll also drink if I'm at a party but I never get invited to parties so it's not really a problem I have to wrestle with. I don't know why this is – is it perhaps because I don't drink so much so am no longer deemed to be fun? Or is it because my social circle is getting smaller as I get older and a lot of my friendships are online with people I've met through Instagram?

My ideal party was back when I was in my teens. The kind where you rock up, get off with loads of boys, vomit in the garden and then eat pizza on the night bus home with your friends. Those days are long gone.

If this isn't what the party is going to be like, then I'll give it a miss.

The ladette culture taught us that drinking was cool

Hands up who was loving the paparazzi pictures of people like Zoe Ball and Sara Cox and Kate Moss rolling out of nightclubs? Hedonism was very cool in the noughties, and the photos of Kate Moss smoking at Glastonbury (I think she had a tin of beer in one hand or looked like she'd been on something heavier) really reiterated that it was cool to drink and that it was right that women had equality and all that jazz. This was also the time when a lot of booze was targeted at women, so when I was at university there were lots of alcopops that tasted really sweet and were easy to glug back and it didn't feel like you were drinking much. At university I ended up sleeping with a singer in a band that was called (don't laugh please) Shooter, and he was called Dobby or maybe Nobby (I can't remember because I was so out of it). Most of the encounters I had with men were fuelled by alcohol and this was another dangerous side of drinking. It made me think that turd-like, crap-merchants were attractive. It made me feel like it was okay to sleep with them. And it was (I'm not being moralistic), but I regretted my choices. It certainly didn't make me cool that I had no standards. (Dobby or Nobby was actually very good-looking, if I remember correctly, and I've tried Googling him many times just to see if he's still around/what he looks like/whether he's got married or not.)

It's no surprise that women coming into their forties and mid-forties and early fifties still feel like drinking is cool and aspirational. Maybe it was fairly aspirational when we were in our twenties, but is it really that cool now we're older? And isn't it a bit limiting to only have booze as an escape from ourselves and the pressures of modern life?

I spoke to Mandy Manners, who has co-written a book with Kate Bailey called *Love Yourself Sober* (see the Resources), which focuses on offering advice for women who want to stay sober. We discussed the challenges of booze and how we need to think about our relationship with it in order to understand whether it's serving us or actually amplifying fears and anxieties (sadly often the latter).

Booze has been made very attractive to women

Mandy explains how women have traditionally been lucrative targets for the alcohol industry:

In the 80s the alcohol industry saw an untapped market and wanted to get women hooked, so romanticised drinking wine and bringing it into the home, and we've seen this happen with the gin market – it was specifically targeted at mums. Then you read around the subject and learn what alcohol does to the brain and how it initially gives you a temporary calming effect by mimicking the neurotransmitter GABA. Therefore, your brain produces less and the next day your brain is lacking in GABA, so you feel even worse. You try to rebalance and end up drinking again and so the vicious cycle begins. It is a depressant and it fuels anxiety. That helped me investigate how I felt about drinking.

She became more aware that whilst booze was a natural choice for much of the female population, it wasn't habitual for everyone and this made her reconsider her own lifestyle:

Alcohol became a social lubricant and stress reliever for me – then I realised that 45 per cent of the world population don't drink alcohol and they are coping with all these things without alcohol. They aren't unhappy people – they don't rely on booze. You have to then think about what you're seeking. Is it stress relief? There are other ways to do that without the after-effects. It becomes so narrow. It's a drug and that's its job.

Drunk women are more fun, yes?

When I was growing up, one of my favourite programmes was *Absolutely Fabulous*. In fact, when I got to adulthood I was somewhat disappointed to realise that grown-ups didn't live in enormous houses with fridges full of booze. I loved Edina Monsoon and Patsy Stone (and still do) and the fact that they spent every waking hour getting pissed and having adventures. I grew up always thinking booze was fun and looked forward to getting pissed when I got to their age. And part of that has stayed with me – the idea that you can't have adventures and fun unless you drink. I had the same relationship with smoking. I used to think it was cool and made you look like a rock star, but now when I see people puffing away on a fag, I think it looks rather sad and lonely. Nonetheless, the idea that sober people are boring and not great to hang out with is pervasive in society. Sometimes when you tell a friend that you've stopped drinking you feel like there's a post-it note on your head saying 'Boring old twat' and nobody wants to hang out with you anymore.

Mandy explains more about how getting drunk isn't always a shortcut to fun:

> When we're young, we don't have responsibilities. But when you get older, then you know *Ab Fab* isn't really a fantasy state and maybe there's more to life than reliving your youth. Since I stopped drinking, I've realised a shit party is a shit party. I have been to a couple of weddings sober and one of them was rubbish because I didn't know the people very well or have much in common and felt obliged to be there and it wasn't fun. I would have usually drunk to excess to make it go away – a free bar is dangerous for anyone who grew up binge-drinking. Funnily enough, I learnt that I have become less serious without booze. I was stuck in thinking I must keep alcohol in my life because it's normal – there was a lot of control and it's tiring to think about drinking/not drinking or not drinking too much all the time, and so when I stopped I began to be more silly and not take myself so seriously.

It took a while for Mandy to realise that being sober was the best route forward for her:

> We [Mandy and her husband] gave up for six months and I loved it because I didn't know you could enjoy mornings. Then I got pregnant and had kids. I started drinking again. Motherhood switched things for me. I'd had a traumatic experience at eighteen and hid this away and hoped it would go away. One of the reasons women drink is often trauma and 'Me too' experiences. I was terrified something would happen to my daughter, and I have PTSD [post-traumatic stress disorder]. It was just lots of things. Living in France, I would get lonely and would have big parties

with my friends, then I was getting overwhelmed and would get really angry with my kids and I'd drink to calm down and feel shit. It was a negative cycle. I was blacking out and waking up at four in the morning and then saying I wouldn't drink. Then by 6pm the next day I would and then I'd feel shit about myself. My self-esteem was really low. So, I decided to quit for a year and loved it. I quit my job and then I started drinking again as I felt so much better and thought I had proved I didn't have a problem. I just made different rules – not drinking on my own. Not drinking during the week, but it still made me unhappy.

I look up to women like Mandy who have chosen sobriety. I am currently in a bit of a limbo. I drink occasionally but don't fully enjoy it, especially if I have one too many, and I find that overall, the after-effects don't make it worth my while. Why haven't I gone sober then? I think the problem is that I am still a little bit in love with the idea of alcohol. I don't have many vices left and there is a childish part of me that feels I need to hold onto a tiny glimmer of rebellion. I know on a rational level that booze isn't cool but I can't quite wave goodbye to it forever. So, for now I am open and curious and fully aware that I feel better without alcohol in my life but am not yet ready to give it up forever. Like many people I also found myself upping my alcohol consumption during Covid-19 – justifying it because I was stuck in a work/no childcare/high anxiety/we're all going to die/I've just lost my dad conundrum. I quickly realised that stepping up my gin intake didn't help, and cut back again. As I've already said, alcohol these days is more likely to push me into the dark side. This is exacerbated by the fact that my dad had problems with alcohol which worsened towards the end of his life. This means that again I have felt the need to rethink the way I have used it – in effect, to numb pain and past trauma.

But should we continue drinking if it's not a problem?

Mandy talks about a 'grey area' when we justify drinking because we think we have it under control and we have a healthy enough relationship with it. So, we think about Nicholas Cage in the film *Leaving Las Vegas* drinking neat vodka in the morning as a problem; or driving drunk, or *Ab Fab* and waking up in a skip as a problem (but it's funny); but what if it's just wine now and then?

Mandy elaborates further:

> To define problematic drinking The World Health Organisation talks about alcohol use disorder. Hazardous drinking is drinking over the recommended units, but there is no external harm. The next level is harmful drinking and there are a lot of people doing that. Drinking over the recommended units and experiencing negative effects like poor mental health, blackouts and/or binge drinking. Then the final category would be alcohol dependant – a strong desire to consume: you have trouble controlling drinking and it impacts on your life in a significant manner.

A lot of people probably fall into the 'harmful' category without really realising it. It's worthwhile thinking about when and how you consume alcohol and whether you want to take a break. Mandy recommends that ideally you should aim to be sober for three months and then see how you feel and what alternatives you could use to address stress and anxiety. This might be having a hot bath or watching a film or going for a run or listening to music on your headphones really loud. There is a myriad of ways to 'treat' yourself that don't involve alcohol.

Personally, I notice that when I'm not drinking, I have less anxiety. Less anger and less ranting. I am a nicer person. If someone hands me a drink, then I'm basically Keith Richards. I tend to indulge in other hedonistic behaviours like smoking Vogue

Menthols, and maybe even doing other illicit substances (though, to be fair, I can't remember the last time I took any drugs).

The thing is that women are under enormous pressure. The year 2020 has taught us that we often shoulder a lot of the emotional strain. It's women who have tended to manage home-schooling; it's women who have been more vulnerable to losing their jobs; it's women who have done the lion's share of domestic admin (so were probably up late at night trying to organise a Tesco delivery). Thinking about these stressors and then adding a layer of menopausal hormones and then not being outside as much or having access to support networks and then drowning all of this with wine and gin… Well, it's easy to see why it's not going to help women long term.

If we are under prolonged periods of stress, then we need to find more sustainable ways to get through, and unfortunately drinking a lot isn't going to work.

For me the following equation is not ideal:

Booze + peri-menopause + young kids + desire to build a career + write + sleep properly + not argue with partner for no reason = not possible.

Awful things that can happen when you're pissed

Whenever I am bored of being sober and am thinking about what a sad sap I am as I stare into my fizzy water (with a slice of cucumber and ice to make it more EXCITING), I try and recall some of the terrible things that can happen when you're drunk. This list is not a list of things I have done (well some of them are) but are gleaned from stories about other people I know being pissed. It helps to realise that it's not always glamorous and it can actually be pretty tawdry and shameful too.

Saying bad things

You're more likely to say something you shouldn't. As much as I love the idea of being more honest as you get older, and not giving a fuck and all that stuff that you read in the standard Renée Zellweger interview, being really boozed up can also result in saying some things that you can't take back again. AND ONCE THE CAT IS OUT OF THE BAG YOU CAN'T SHOVE THAT HAIRY MONSTER BACK IN AGAIN.

Having accidents

Accidents happen. These can obviously be super-dangerous accidents but there are also the kind that don't actually kill you but are nonetheless awful anyway. The husband of one of my friends tried to get his hands out of his pockets whilst exiting a bar and instead fell straight onto the concrete pavement with his face and knocked all his teeth out. He went to bed and didn't think anything of it until he woke up like old man Steptoe and had to spend thousands on emergency dental surgery. (Is this cool and exciting? Methinks not.)

Being a horrible lech

Sometimes your flirty side comes out. Having a crush on a dad at the school gates is one thing (am I the only person who gets this?), but actually sidling up to that dad at some boring function and breathing all over him and trying to seduce him in a not very subtle way IS NOT a good look. I haven't done this by the way but I have definitely thought about it and luckily was at an 'International Food Cuisine Celebration' in the school hall and there was no booze available so I remained sitting on a tiny school chair munching samosas and not making eye contact with the dad in question, so was okay.

Looking after children is not advisable

I am ashamed to say that there have been times when I've been in charge of kids and under the influence. I have found it terrifying, to be frank (not in the moment itself but the following day). I have tried to steer a buggy home whilst unable to see straight and have gone through the bedtime routine like a zombie – just willing myself to get through and everyone to be okay so I can collapse on the floor. I'm not proud of this. I don't want my kids to remember me being pissed up and swaying about whilst trying to get their legs into their pyjamas. I also don't buy into the whole 'drinking mothers is a very cool thing' and think there is a lot of pressure on women to booze. Sometimes we need to think about other avenues that make us feel better longer term. If you're getting shit-faced at every opportunity, then you have to question what's going wrong with your life. Are you bored? Are you frustrated? Is there anything else you can do that is slightly less hazardous? And let me say that I've been there. I have been the mother so drunk that I had to have someone help me out the door (and I almost tripped) and I now think about all the things that could have happened but luckily didn't, perhaps because of the manifesting I talked about in the previous chapter.

A tribute to Kate Moss

Basically, if you're a woman in your mid-forties, then Kate Moss was quite likely your style icon for some time. I first spotted her in *The Face* magazine when I was about seventeen and living in Amsterdam. I was quite spaced out, for various reasons, and used to make collages by cutting up magazines and sticking things together. I made a lovely collage of Kate – she was standing astride a mountain and everyone was looking up at her with worshipful gazes. Then I came back to London and she was going out with Johnny Depp (who isn't an aspirational heart throb nowadays for a myriad of reasons but he was back in the day).

Kate and I shared so many similarities. We'd grown up in South London and I'd gone to Sydenham Girls and she'd been just up the road in Croydon and she was spotted by a model scout when she was a teenager and my best friend Amy was also spotted by a model scout (this was where our stories changed a bit) and Kate always seemed to have a weakness for musicians or actors and I did too (but usually they didn't have the hots for me). Then our paths really went in totally different directions as I embarked on a career in market research and talking to people about peas and whether they liked pea packaging or not and she flew all over the world modelling and going to parties and festivals and looking amazing. I heard debauched stories of how she'd had orgies in hotels and taken loads of drugs, and meanwhile I was usually in the Slug & Lettuce in Notting Hill, eating chunky chips and drinking bottles of white wine. When her fashion range for Top

Shop came out, I bought just about every piece in the collection (I also bought the pirate boots and wore them with mini-skirts, despite being a size 14 with very short legs and looking like an overweight Adam Ant clone).

Kate had so many lovely men in her life. (I wasn't keen on Pete Doherty, though – my friend put it best when she said he'd be sure to have a pongy willy.) I have never actually seen a bad photo of her – even when she was coming out of a club at 3am. Even then. It took me a long time to realise that the clothes Kate wore didn't actually suit normal girls. I wore skinny jeans despite the fact that they were incredibly unflattering on my figure. I based my entire wardrobe on the stuff she wore. I carried on smoking because she was always smoking in every photo I saw of her. Then PUFF, I turned forty and realised that I'd spent much of my entire adult life wishing I was Kate Moss and being obsessive about her life and it wasn't healthy because if it continued, I'd never actually have a life of my own (I also threw out the pirate boots and the concept of me looking great in shorts of any kind).

The truth is Kate Moss was a heroine to many women. She continues to look great today. I salute her but I accept that I am not her.

And I'm just starting (aged forty-seven) to feel okay about that.

Style tips for OLDER women

Did you see the iconic Coronavirus Boris Johnson speech where he kept giving confusing advice like 'Don't go to work, go to work' and 'Take public transport, don't take public transport'? Well, this is how I feel about fashion and the advice that's doled out every couple of months. This is especially true as you get into your forties and start to notice articles about things that are permissible for older women to wear and things that aren't. You know, the ones that say you can't wear mini-skirts and you should show off your arms but only if you work out and have good hands that haven't aged; and if you don't work out, then you should wear a kaftan but not any kaftan, an incredibly expensive one, not one from the Judi Dench range because you're not *that* old but one from another boutique, but don't wear sandals because you're too old for sandals, but you can wear sandals if they're 200 quid and if Victoria Beckham has worn them, but maybe don't wear them because there is nothing worse than old feet/hands/arms/legs/chest, so best not to wear anything or go anywhere because NOBODY WANTS TO SEE A DISGUSTING OLD WOMAN. CAN'T YOU GET THE MESSAGE, YOU TWAT? And do use public transport, don't use public transport.

Those same old, same old trends keep coming. I can repeat verbatim the feature on 'how to dress like Jane Birkin', and whilst I love her, I will never look like her in a million years no matter how hard I try. If you are a size 16 and in your forties the 'waif/gamine' look is a hard one to pull off. A stripey top makes me look like Kirsty Allsop.

Here are some '*anti-tips*' for those of you that hate fashion tips for older women:

- Dungarees are great, as are boilersuits and jumpsuits. In the summer I wear long skirts but can't wear shorts as they make me look like Dennis the Menace.
- If I read one more article about 'the classic white shirt' I will explode. The classic white shirt only exists if you have no children, never come into contact with any mess and are driven by a chauffeur who feeds you latte through a straw to avoid any spillages.
- I dress for women. Men don't notice what you're wearing unless you're dressed in black, rubber hot-pants.
- Wearing draped cardigans ages you, as do linen and kaftans (but it's fine as long as you're aware of that).

- Beware of linen – even if it is hot and summer. Linen is not kind to big arses.
- Give up trying to look like Kate Moss.
- Wear colour. But don't wear colour if you don't like it.
- Stop hunting for the perfect pair of jeans. Do other stuff instead, like volunteering or picking up rubbish in your local park.
- Trainers are a good way of signalling that you still have your hand in fashion-wise.
- Wear clothes that make you happy.
- Beware the 'wacky old lady' fashion thing where you wear bright glasses and earrings and shoes (i.e. Sue Pollard, unless you aspire to be Sue Pollard).
- Do the 'wacky old lady' thing, because frankly, who cares?
- Ditch heels. Or wear them if you like them.
- Ignore all fashion advice.

CHAPTER NINE

How Friendships Get Better with Age

So far, I've learnt that being in your forties is an up and down time with lots of things to think about, but one of the real positives of this time is this: YOU NO LONGER HAVE ANY TOLERANCE FOR CRAP. And this 'no-tolerance for crap' policy means that ultimately your friendships are better than they were when you were younger. I checked in with a few friends recently and this is what they said about how your friendships evolve:

> I have four best friends. We have a WhatsApp group that we use as a daily diary. We see each other probably once a year but we treat the group as a vault/counselling session/pick-me-up/mirror/period tracker, etc.

> As you get older you tread a middle line. You're evolving into a new phase of life so you're a bit insecure again and you want to retain your sense of independence and creativity, but at the same time you want people around you that are grounded and real and who support you implicitly.

> I'm definitely clearer on my own boundaries and that helps detect the bad ones. You just know in your gut. Not always easy to manage, but it's easier than when I was younger. I think because my priorities are so different and I have so little spare time and

energy. Quality of friendships has definitely improved for me as I've got older.

So, you go deeper with your friendships, share more, are better at creating boundaries and rely more on your gut. There may be ups and downs but, overall, there's a sense that the quality of friendships vastly improves as you get older.

Goodbye people pleasing

In my twenties and early thirties I was a classic people pleaser and I wanted everyone to like me. The problem was I wanted them to like me even if I didn't like them. Cue lots of boring drinks in pubs after work, listening to people and pretending to laugh, and going home and trying to analyse every comment they'd made to see if there was any underlying problem they might have with me. I look back on those days now and feel so sad about all the wasted time. Time spent analysing things. Time spent sitting and staring at people and trying to figure out why they might not approve of me. Why hadn't they laughed at that particular joke? Was it not funny or was it offensive in some way? Why had I ended up buying drinks for everyone again? Why had the really unattractive man in the group not fancied me? The thing is, we are socially conditioned as women to want to be liked. We are told from an early age (even if you have feminist parents, you pick it up from the broader culture) that we should be nice and affable and that being bolshy and difficult isn't acceptable. This impacts on your friendships at times, and when you meet people you want their approval. That's not to say I didn't have any meaningful friendships, because I did, but they were often the exception.

Somewhere in my mid-to-late thirties my friendships started to change. I woke up one day and realised I didn't have many friends. Or I did but I rarely saw them anymore. The majority were in the rush hour of bringing up small kids. Basically, I hadn't realised that when you have a baby, then you really want to talk about the baby and so you need other women with babies to do that with. I was still in a high-profile job and spending all my time trying to make myself happy buying Diptique candles and Bella Freud jumpers (sounds like heaven but it wasn't – ironic, hey?). I then embarked on fertility treatment and that's when the nature of friendships really evolved again.

When you're going through something like IVF, then you develop a certain radar for other women on the same level. You want to chat about hormone injections and acupuncture and scans, and the rest of the world fades into the background for a while. I sat in cafés with other women undergoing treatment, and five minutes in we'd be talking about the size of our uterus or how our eggs were doing. The bonding was intense. I learnt that intense and meaningful friendships can spring out of misery and that you can attract the people you need in that particular time. The shittiness of the situation intensifies everything. Your basic conversations go something like this: 'Listen up, let's cast aside the competitive shit and who has the biggest house, and let's just get down and talk about our real feelings.'

So, one of the things you learn is that through sharing vulnerability and being really honest with others, you can make deep connections. This vulnerability is important and for me is a litmus test of a good friendship. If people don't respond to be being open and honest about the stuff I'm going through, if they make me feel bad or guilty for opening up… Well, I know they're not really my cup of tea. That doesn't mean that I get free licence to bore everyone to death but it does mean I want to have really honest and authentic relationships, otherwise I'd rather not bother at all. I have spent enough time skirting on the surface, making chit-chat about the weather.

The older you are, the better and more authentic your friendships become

Fast forward to today and I have a very clear idea of what kind of people make good friends. I also don't care (so much) about what people think about me. I can weed out the people that will be good pals and I stay away from those who won't. I don't mean to sound cruel, but the truth is I don't want to feel crap. My life is often crap – like everyone's it contains challenges and issues – and so I don't need friends who amplify that crap. I only have a finite amount of time left. The fact that my dad died recently has only reminded me of that. I am fairly good at beating myself up and making myself feel bad, so I don't need a friend to do this – unless I'm out of line and have done something that needs calling out. I wish I could say that I no longer stay awake at night analysing what people think of me. What I would say, though, is that I spend less time on that stuff than before (instead I worry about ageing, my kids, pandemics, climate change, where all the school cardigans have gone, when I'll find a job I actually enjoy, if I'll ever have sex again – that kind of thing).

I am ruthless with my friendships in many ways. Just like back in my IVF days, I feel things in my gut. I don't make people fill in a questionnaire or anything, I just know. Many of my friendships are nurtured in the local park whilst the kids are playing. I have made great friends in the park. I don't hang back if I like someone, and I try to make it as obvious as possible. Okay, this is risky as it can make you look desperate, but frankly I *am* desperate. I'm desperate to make connections with people that I feel an affinity with. So, if I get the odd knock-back, then that's okay. I don't have a huge friendship circle – not the kind of circle I had in my twenties, anyway (but these were all going-out friends and we hadn't much in common) – but the friends that I do have now are precious.

Friendships aren't just about ME, ME, ME

There has been a lot of chat on social media about how some people are 'radiators' and others 'drains', and I've definitely noticed that there are some women who I walk away from after a conversation and I need a lie-down. Yes, I feel drained. Having said that, I worry that we're becoming too self-orientated when it comes to friendships. There are going to be times when you find relationships draining. There will be times when friends are going through challenges and need your support. There are times when I'm aware that I'm a real DRAG. I am incredibly self-obsessed and don't listen enough. I am too busy thinking about the next thing to say rather than really listening to the other person.

However, you can't build a friendship circle out of people who solely plump up your ego and make you feel good. If we only want friends that are positive and 'radiate good vibes', then we end up with a bunch of gurning chimps, not real people with ups and downs. We end up like Kim Kardashian with a group of personal assistants who are likely to do everything she wants (sometimes I fantasise about what this would be like and have come to the conclusion that to begin with it's fun but long term it must make you fed up – the fact that nobody tells you the truth). One worrying thing I've noticed is that I lack a lot of mental bandwidth when it comes to friendships. I have a nagging feeling that I need to be more supportive but feel too depleted to offer much. This may be because I'm still grieving for my dad, or it may be the ripple effect of Covid-19 and parenting small kids and cats that won't give me a minute's peace… but it's something I'm aware I want to work on. I am aware that friends don't exist on this planet to blow smoke up my arse.

Recently a friend critiqued some writing I'd done and I felt furious. My initial reaction was to stop speaking to her. This rang alarm bells once I'd calmed down. I realised that my ego was inflated and she had a point. I needed to listen to her but my knee-jerk response was to say, 'OFF WITH HER HEAD!' This comes down to the whole idea of rigidity versus growth – as we age, we can become one of those people who is very quick to judge others. I realised that the reason I was hurt was because I was feeling insecure and I needed to be open and tell her that. One of the other downsides of social media is that we are so quick to respond and do so without thinking. We scroll through our feeds and go *like, like, like*; and we size people up and go *like, like*… no wait… *don't like*. We see people as images that we size up in a second, versus complex individuals with conflicting opinions and ups and downs. In real life, things are more subtle and complex. We can have things we don't like about our friends and they can give us home truths. They can be right arseholes and yet we need to live with that or we are essentially having superficial relationships and nothing deeper.

I have noticed on social media that people tend to block others the minute they disagree with them or say something provocative, and then I think, hang on, is there no room for disagreement? Is there no room for difficult people? Or needy people? Do we just want to give 'thumbs up' emojis all day long? And if we are sad and needy and anxious, then does that mean we should be avoided? This isn't a question that I've resolved yet. I think, in theory, I like people who challenge me, call me out if I'm being rude or judgemental and expand the way I think about the world. I might not like them in the moment but when I get time to sit down and think about it, I don't want to only have friends that are nice and 'radiate' 24/7 because then I'd probably think something was up with them and they weren't really being honest and authentic.

I hope my friends feel they can be honest with me. I hope they'll call me out if I'm acting like a wanker. I don't mind if they are sometimes drains, because I am sometimes a drain too. I am aware that I need to get better at being a good friend – in the same way that I work at being a better parent.

Why it's important to SEE friends and not just send them emojis

In this modern age with multiple communication channels on your phone and lots of tabs open in your head, there's a danger that you stop seeing friends. It can simply feel too exhausting. It's easier surely to just ping off a message and move onto the next task of the day? Friends can feel like another thing 'to do', and so arranging to meet face to face and then having a proper conversation… Well isn't it just too much? This isn't necessarily an age thing of course. In 2020 we didn't see people anyway. Or we only saw them with certain rules in place. The thing is, YOU DO NEED TO ACTUALLY SEE YOUR FRIENDS. Sending them a text or a giphy from *Schitt's Creek* is all well and good but if you don't see them in the flesh, then you're not likely to have the same kind of messy, up-and-down, interesting relationship. It gets a bit like a game of *kissy kissy ping pong* – you send a message, they send a message, you bat one back, they bat one back – you start to build up this sense that you can just communicate with everyone this way. It's dangerous. I recently tried to send a text message to my daughter who is two. I realised that my brain was only thinking in messages. Short message and emoji. Short message and emoji. *Kissy kissy ping pong.* Then you finally see the person in the flesh and you're like WOW. This is what a friendship is. I can see their eyes. I can touch their arm (when we're no longer socially distancing that is). We can cry. We can hug. Tech is great. It's fab. It is no replacement for seeing the people you love. It just isn't.

So, here's a quick quiz so you can tell whether a friend is really a proper friend. Ask yourself the following ten questions:

1. Do you look forward to seeing them?
2. Do you laugh together?
3. Would you let them see your house in a bit of a state?
4. Would you reveal a vulnerability about yourself?
5. Do you find it easy to talk to them?
6. If something happens in your life, do you get the urge to contact them immediately to let them know?
7. Would you cry in front of them?
8. Do they inspire you?
9. Do they encourage you to do new things?
10. Do you miss them when you don't see them?

If you answer 'yes' to at least six of these, then they are the kind of friend that will help you navigate ageing and all the other ups and downs that life throws our way. If you answer 'no', then maybe rethink what you get out of this relationship. If it's just a mutual love of taxidermy and browsing vintage markets, then that's okay too…

One of the biggest things I've missed since losing my dad was not having any friends to hug me. I had lots of lovely texts. I got cards. I got flowers. I was lucky. The thing was, I couldn't get hugs from friends because there was a pandemic. Of course, I got them from my partner and my kids, but when I finally met up with friends it was weird because we couldn't touch. I realised that a big part of friendship is the physical side. Put quite simply, I can't wait to hug my friends again.

So, what is my final piece of advice about friendship in your forties and fifties?

Cherish it. It's precious. And when you get the opportunity, hug. And listen. Show your vulnerability. And don't just rely on your phone to keep in touch. Prioritise seeing them.

I will have friends who are reading this now and thinking, 'She's talking a load of guff. I haven't seen her in yonks.' And they're right. And I'm going to sort that out.

I promise.

CHAPTER TEN

Don't You Want Me Baby?

Why Ageing Isn't That Sexy but Should Be

Once I passed forty, MEN NO LONGER LOOKED AT ME. Okay, I'm exaggerating. It wasn't men, it was men under the age of seventy-five. Suddenly I became a honey trap for any ageing blokes over that age but I was invisible to every other male.

It wasn't subtle. Some old men would roll their window down so they could stick their 'special-sold-in-the-back-of-the-*Daily-Mail*-magnifying-glass' out and get a better look at me. It was overwhelming. In the pub. In the Londis. In the local park as they leched over the fence. I was catnip for the Two Ronnies brigade. As a forty-year-old I was seriously being assessed as fair game. I'd entered a stage where men my dad's age thought I was sexy. It was sad. It made me feel like my life was over. I have nothing against old(er) men. I'm not so keen on the ones that shout, 'HEY, LOVE, FANCY SOME DOGGING?' out their van window, but I'm happy to chat to anyone really. The main problem is I don't want to sleep with a seventy-eight-year-old man. (Maybe Mick Jagger – is he seventy-eight? I'd be curious to see what all the fuss is about, but I'm not a Brazilian supermodel so don't hold out much hope.) The thing is, if I think it's not okay for old men to lech at me, then isn't it also wrong for me to lech after men that are 15–20 years younger than me? Isn't it double standards otherwise?

The thing is, I'm not immune to the odd crush on a younger man. If *I* think it's okay, then it should be okay for old men to lust after *me*, right? I recently watched a Harry Styles performance at an awards show and found myself thinking inappropriate thoughts and realised that Harry 'Hunky Sizzler' Styles (I've made that middle name up – sort of like a *Just 17* caption – sorry) was born in 1994. In that year I'd just embarked on a degree in media studies, had cropped white hair, wore combat trousers and was drinking Hooch in large quantities. I could have easily given birth to Styles but wouldn't have been a good mum as I went out every night and had a weakness for Northern men with feather cuts. So, is it socially acceptable for me to think about Harry in this way?

I wasn't the only forty-something woman watching *Normal People*, the Sally Rooney TV drama, and crushing on Connell Waldron played by Paul Mescal. Of course, it wasn't just the way he looked; it was also his sensitivity and his complex, nuanced character (but it was also the way he looked – of course it was).

If a man is forty-seven and has a twenty-four-year-old girlfriend, I'll think, 'OH YES, MIDLIFE-CRISIS-LAND'. But is it okay if it's the other way round? (So, female artist Sam Taylor Johnson has a husband, Aaron Taylor Johnson, and she's fifty-three and he's thirty – that seems acceptable to many – me included.) But the thing is, do you remember the TV comedy show *Shooting Stars* with Vic Reeves and Bob Mortimer? The vision of Vic Reeves lasciviously rubbing his knees at whatever female guest was on that week. It feels a bit lecherous. A bit wrong. Or maybe it's empowering as it's obviously something men have been doing since the dawn of time. A few years ago, I was drunk at a work party and a young guy was chatting to me about something and I thought I'd try and impress him by telling him I'd once hung out with Kim Deal from *The Breeders*. (This is true. I did.)

'Who's the Breeders?' he asked, shrugging.

'Are you seriously telling me that you haven't heard of Kim Deal?' I said, the vein in my ageing neck popping out.

'Never heard of him.'

I walked off feeling ancient. I also realised that I'd struggle dating a much younger man. He wouldn't get any of my cultural reference points, and most of the music I listen to grinds to a halt in 2001. (I still feel like the 80s and 90s were the best time music-wise, however much I try and learn about new bands.)

Anyway, so okay, the younger man is off-limits for me, and I have a partner and he's actually ten years older than me. We have been together a long time and we've had (like most couples) good and bad times. Like many in long-term relationships, we've probably questioned why we're together but then re-evaluated and realised that there are more pros than cons and we still get a lot of joy out of one another.

The only problem is sex. Or lack of sex. Or highly infrequent sex. Today when I read articles about people in retirement villages and homes getting lots of STDs because they're bonking one another senseless, there is part of me that thinks, 'YES, YOU GO THERE, DUDES! WHY NOT?' Another part of me knows it's not for me. When I'm in my eighties, I definitely want to waft about in a long nightie, watch re-runs of *Line of Duty* and eat crab-paste sandwiches (I'm looking forward to this time, which will also be the time when I'll take up smoking again, possibly cigars). I feel like NOW should be the time when I'm having the best sex of my life. But I'm not. And why not? Because I'm tired. Because there are so many other things to do. Because I'm in a long-term relationship and we probably take one another for granted. Because I put it off. Because I want to watch TV and zonk out at the end of the day.

The problem is that if I leave sex and never have it again, then my entire life has been a mixed bag – sex-wise (which let's be honest, is probably true for most women).

My not very sexy history from teens to today

My teens

Really good levels of snogging, and a bit of terrible sex because I didn't know what the heck was going on. I had zero self-esteem and didn't have good judgement when it came to the opposite sex. I was also experimenting with alcohol, which chiefly meant drinking a bottle of Thunderbird Red and then vomiting all over the place and repeating that experiment each week. I developed crushes on emotionally unavailable men who wore too much aftershave and had perms. (Al, you know you broke my heart, right?) Essentially, like many teenage women, the more someone ignored me and was mean, the more I thought they were interesting and someone with long-term potential. If they didn't call when they said they would (and this was before mobiles and you had to hit 1471 to check if you'd missed calls), I would fall head over heels with them. It spelt mystery and intrigue and all sorts of good stuff to me.

My twenties

I was in a long-term relationship and the sex was good to begin with. It was an intense relationship – one of those that you often have in your late teens/early twenties, but I still very much saw sex as something that happened to me, that I had no control of, that I couldn't shape or give direction to. I developed a lot of crushes during this period but never had the courage to tell the people I had crushes on that I had crushes on them. I observed a lot of quite rampant behaviour sex-wise, but was usually the one in the background trying to find the coffee pot/vacuum/sugar bowl. I was usually the one trying to inject normality into the situation.

My thirties

Sex with my long-term partner was great but it was also erratic
because I was super-stressed, prioritising work and then became
obsessed with getting pregnant. I also continued the theme
developed in my childhood – the theme of not feeling great about
my body, and so this became a barrier. I preferred to have sex with
the lights off and under a duvet, which restricted the number of
positions I could trial and took a fair amount of joy away from
the experience. Fertility treatment is not an aphrodisiac either and
can take away any sense of pleasure – your body becomes a thing
that is broken and isn't working properly, and the hormones and
stress didn't help my low libido.

My forties

With two small children, intimacy has now slipped to the bottom
of the list of things to do. Also, I feel shit about my body because
everything is drooping and I don't want anyone to see it, even my
partner who I have been with for twenty plus years. I know that
I should feel better/do more/make it a priority, but the reality is
that I haven't (but I will get round to it eventually).

I have always felt that if my sex life was a school report, then
it would say in big red biro: *ANNIKI COULD DO BETTER.*

I've always been inhibited but have been in a few debauched
situations through the years and have had friends who have been
into S&M. I've co-hosted a podcast all about sex and relationships
whilst I rarely have sex at all. I've had friends who have been
polygamous. Friends who frequent sex parties. I have listened to
them with curiosity but have been too scared to try any of these
things. (I did, however, make a film at university about S&M
and there were aspects that appealed – especially the fact that you

could get submissive people to clean your house for you. This is something I've filed away as I hate cleaning.)

For me, poor body image is a barrier and I've grown up seeing my body as the enemy – an ugly thing that didn't do what I wanted it to. I was overweight as a child. I've always hated my thick, short legs, so I've tended to avoid any positions that involved someone seeing them (which is actually pretty much impossible if you think about it). I also hate my stomach, and this has got worse over time (and I'm trying to say positive affirmations – believe me) and so try to avoid positions that show that off too. This means that I can only really choose positions that showcase my arms and neck (oh, and my face), which is quite limiting in terms of delving into the Kama Sutra and styling things out.

So what can we do if we're unhappy with our current sex lives?

I've met women in the past who are comfortable in their bodies. They will happily strip off in a gym changing room, whatever their size. I feel like the comments in my childhood and being called 'FATTY BOOM BOOM' (usually accompanied by the song of the same name) in the playground have made it hard to feel great about my physique. I can acknowledge that it's amazing – that I've had two marvellous kids – but I still pretty much hate it most days. This has now been combined with my negative self-talk around ageing and my body. When I get out of the shower, I often recall the scene in *Game of Thrones* when Melisandre – The Red Queen –morphs into an ancient naked woman revealing that she is in fact several thousands of years old. The sad thing is, I've read enough books and blogs to know that I shouldn't feel bad about my body, that it's the patriarchy, that it's ageism, and the fact that all women are judged on their physical selves more than their brain or mental capacities, but I can't escape the feeling that I'd just be happier if I had longer legs and was a size 10.

I've been waiting to hit my sexual peak and it's never happened (perhaps I missed it when I lived in Amsterdam – certainly the opportunities were there). But here I am today. Living in suburban London with a proper job, two small kids, a long-term partner and a desire to try and make my sex life better but also a sense that I don't know where to start. I talked to Dr Karen Gurney who is a Clinical Psychologist and Psychosexologist and Director at The Havelock Clinic. There are complex dynamics going on when it comes to women and ageing and sex and I wanted to get advice on what could be done. She told me:

> Concerns about body image are always a tricky one for women. In fact, it's the number one distraction for women during sex that interferes with their arousal and pleasure. There's a few things to consider here. It may be worth focusing on creating change in how you feel about your body, so that those thoughts don't pop up as much. This might be doing something which makes your body feel good and you know has improved your body confidence before, or it may be from flooding your social media feeds with more body positive accounts.

She acknowledges that the imagery around us is often to blame for the way we relate to our own bodies:

> Our negative ideas about our body come from the constant barrage of 'perfect' bodies we see in the media. The great thing about social media, is for the first time we can curate what we see – so use it! If you've worked on both of these things and still find your mind wanders during sex to what your thighs look like from that angle, then I can really recommend you look into a mindfulness programme for sex.

She says mindfulness can help us come out of our heads and back into our physical senses instead:

> Mindfulness helps you put your attention where you want it, not where you don't. It's been proven in research to help women be more orgasmic, increase desire and keep their attention on what's hot, not on negative thoughts. It's also worth knowing that women's body confidence tends to improve with age, so we've all got something to look forward to there!

But what if you feel stuck in a rut and like you aren't experimental enough in terms of your sex life? Often in long-term relationships we tend to keep having sex in the same way (if we're having it all). Karen feels it's important to try different things and be open to changing the dynamic and kind of sex you have as a couple:

> Often in long-term relationships I find that it's the habits that couples fall into that start to limit them, as if you've only had slow tender sex for fifteen years it can feel so difficult to ask (or do) something different. But I work with many people who say to me, 'I wish they'd just grab me and kiss me sometimes, but they never would.'

So, we may secretly fantasise about having a different kind of sex (not just sex with Harry Styles, for example) but feel unable to bring that novelty into our relationship when novelty is exactly what we need (and possibly why we're fantasising about Harry in the first place). Karen adds:

> The truth is, we are all different people sexually on different days, and we need to be able to play those different roles. The good news is that if you feel stuck in a rut, you can change the culture

of your relationship slowly by bringing a little bit of newness in. My advice is to bring a few (small) things in each year, that you each suggest you do differently.

She also advises that you talk about sex (this is hard, especially if you are zonked out in front of Netflix most evenings, which let's face it, many of us are):

> The best way to normalise this is to have a yearly sexual relationship MOT conversation where you talk about what's going well and what you'd like more of. You would do this with work/your diet/ the kids, so why should sex be any different? These changes don't need to be nipple tassles. It could be spending one evening a month just kissing for hours and nothing else, or banning penetrative sex to every other time you're sexual together, but it will mean that your sex life is always changing, not stagnating.

Karen also says women need to be empowered and educate themselves more:

> I would say you need to learn about how desire works. It's totally different to everything you've been sold, and knowing this will give you all the tools you need to have the sex life that you want, no matter how long you've been together.

And, yes, tiredness and overwhelm can be a big barrier but it can't be used as an excuse not to take action – or not forever anyway. Karen says:

> Tiredness is a big barrier to feeling like sex and shouldn't be sniffed at! You have three options here. The first is to address the tiredness directly (i.e. find a way to get more sleep!). The second is to accept that tiredness is affecting your sex life and one day

you'll get sleep again and don't worry about it for now (this is my advice for new parents). The last one is to accept that tiredness will always be a part of life and schedule time to trigger desire when your tiredness will not be so bad, avoiding times like late at night. The other thing about sex and tiredness is that having sex is a bit like exercising in that you may not feel like it to start off with, but once you've got yourself into that headspace, you really start to enjoy it and the tiredness fades away.

All of this advice makes sense. I've talked to Karen a lot at events and in person, and I've always found that if I do incorporate her tips into my life, my relationship improves. I've become more aware that when I talk to my partner it is often super-functional chat about picking up kids or dinner. This isn't sexy. I am trying to change that and carve out a bit of time when I talk to him as a living, breathing human. I've also found that mindfulness has helped me be more in the moment and stop living in my head. I'm increasingly aware that my sex life won't fix itself. This doesn't mean you have to have sex a certain number of times a year to be deemed 'okay', but if you feel like your sex life isn't great, then it's good to try and think about why that is and slowly move towards a state which is more satisfying.

Oh, and fantasising about younger men is okay, *but* don't let this be a replacement for actually being physical with a real person (i.e. your partner, unless your partner is Harry Styles, that is *eyes glaze over momentarily as Anniki dreams about a scenario where Harry has just come off stage and is slightly sweaty, etc.*).

Sometimes it's the men we thought about when we were younger that stick in our brains as fantasy fodder. I find that, aside from Harry Styles and Cillian Murphy, I've tended to stick with more old-school crushes and not moved on. There's no shame in not updating your roll-call of fantasy men. Nobody can see inside your head and shout that you're not being relevant or need to watch more up-to-date content. Some of these men are no longer around, unfortunately; but if it's a fantasy, then it doesn't actually matter, so fill your boots.

1. Michael Hutchence

I mention Michael a lot in the book Lisa Williams and I wrote, called *More Orgasms Please*, because he still plays on my mind. I sometimes think that if you were trying to design a man with a lot of sex appeal then this is what you'd end up with. I recently watched a documentary all about him (*Mystify*, directed by Richard Lowenstein) and was immediately transported back to being twelve years old and completely obsessed with the man. I try and focus very much on the years that he was with Kylie (so, I am in the Kylie role and this is the great thing about fantasy – I CAN ACTUALLY BE KYLIE IN MY MIND, EVEN THOUGH WE HAVE NO PHYSICAL SIMILARITIES AT ALL, OF COURSE).

2. Dave Grohl

I have a complex fantasy about Dave Grohl. It's not just sex as I think he's also a very funny and intuitive person. So, when I think about him, we're married and I'm living in this incredible mansion in Los Angeles, and Dave spends a lot of time in his music studio, but I'll lounge by the pool whilst the children are taken care of by a lovely nanny (who is also hideously ugly), and the fantasy doesn't actually involve sex because I don't see Dave that way. Instead, he's laughing at my jokes and being really attentive when I tell him my new book ideas, and the main gist is that this is a man that places me at the centre of his universe and uses me as his muse and inspiration. I also get to hang out with all his cool friends, like Josh Homme from Queens of the Stone Age (who is mentioned below), and there is quite a bit of tension between Dave and Josh because they are both in love with me, and yet are also best friends so don't want to talk about it. I have a whole fantasy sequence which involves them both watching me on stage (because I've taken up playing the drums and am excellent at it) and Dave and Josh have the following conversation about me:

> **Josh:** God, she's brilliant – so enigmatic and natural.
>
> **Dave:** Steady on. That's my wife you're talking about.
>
> **Josh:** I feel like the older she's got, the more attractive she is, right?
>
> **Dave:** I didn't really get how good she was at drumming. I mean we're both good, right, but she's kind of blowing us out of the water right now.
>
> **Josh:** She reminds me of a young Janis Joplin.
>
> **Dave:** No, not Janis. Someone more refined. Someone really cool. Anyway, like I said, she's my wife – in fact, I've written a beautiful song all about her which I'm going to play to you later.

Josh: That's a weird coincidence because I've written a song about her too.

[Starting to get pissed off with one another now.]

Dave: Right, well, I'll go and get us a cider, okay? It feels like the mood has got a bit awkward…

3. Josh Homme

I've already mentioned him above, but when I'm not thinking about Dave Grohl, then I'm thinking about this man. I sometimes do a variation on the 'Dave and Josh watching me playing drums' fantasy, and Josh is watching me on his own and I'm singing like Laura Marling (and he's marvelling at my composition skills instead of drumming) and I look like I did when I was eighteen (there was a window in time when everything fell into place but I didn't realise it back then, of course). Josh is entranced by my vocals and can't take his eyes off me. After I've come off stage, he buys me a hot dog with all the trimmings, and then takes me for a ride on his vintage motorcycle and we hang out in the Hollywood Hills. (Again, I don't fantasise about sex. It's more about him being entranced by my talent and not being able to stop staring.) Sometimes I prefer the Dave Grohl combination fantasy as I have both of them arguing over me (something that did actually happen when I was in my early twenties but it was two different men and I was in a bar in Covent Garden and I had terrible hair extensions which fell on the floor during the fight).

4. Brad Pitt

Obvious I know, but I just think he becomes better with age. In my Brad Pitt fantasy I mix things up and am dancing on stage and it's the early 90s or something and he is totally spaced out but asks if I want a drink, and then we dance to some classic dance track like 'You've Got the Love' and he has his arm around me and we're sweaty but also totally chilled and in love.

5. John Taylor

Yes, the bass player from Duran Duran. When I was growing up I was obsessed with John Taylor and used to write letters to the fan club and do terrible drawings of him. I even posed on a climbing frame in my pedal-pusher jumpsuit and mullet hairstyle (I think I had turquoise mascara too) and sent the photo in one of my letters. If I wrote a letter to John now it would go something like this:

Dear John,

I just Googled to see a recent image of you (this is obviously not the first time I've done this) and you are still a 'chod' (this is what I called a HUNK back in the day). I don't know if you received the letters I wrote – it would have been around 1984, and I guess you didn't keep the photograph of me on the climbing frame because it felt wrong. I didn't look great in pedal-pushers, and I think you were dating a German supermodel. I had braces on my teeth, and spots where I'd shaved my eyebrows off with my dad's razor – I did enter some modelling competitions but my rugby player legs got in the way of a career on the catwalk. You then had it off with Amanda de Cadenet, who I sort of looked up to because she was always at glamorous parties in the newspapers. I was in a Dutch house act in Amsterdam just after that time and can't remember very much apart from eating a lot of chips and smoking huge quantities of fags and trying to make some cash cleaning music studios. (I met

Lenny Kravitz once and Vince Clarke from Erasure worked downstairs – do you know them? I always think all famous musicians must hang out.)

Anyway, the fact that we never went out with one another makes me sad, but I also realise that I was in love with an idea. Like many crushes it was the idea of a perfect man that doesn't exist. I was objectifying you and didn't acknowledge that you were a really talented bass player (I did buy *The Power Station* album, though, even though none of my friends had heard of it, and thought the lead singer Robert Palmer was a creepy grandad – I also fancied him, by the way, but I fancied you much more).

Anyway, one day our paths will cross. Maybe on Oprah, but I suspect you're not into late forty-something women in boilersuits. I can send you a photo of me today if you like. I left having children very late, so my body isn't quite supermodel standard. We wouldn't have sex anyway, but I'd be happy to snog you for a couple of hours?

All the best,
Anniki

CHAPTER ELEVEN

All the Awful Shit Like Death, Grief and Facing Up to Your Own Mortality

I've saved one of the worst things that ever happened to me for this chapter. When I was fifteen, I lost my step-mum and sister.

Janine, my step-mum was suffering with severe post-partum psychosis and jumped off a tower block with my baby sister in her arms. My sister Frances was five months old. It was the kind of shock that reverberates for years and neither my dad nor I recovered. I rarely talk about it as I find it's an instant buzz-killer – people don't know how to respond to someone who's grieving and if the circumstances are somewhat extraordinary and sad, then that becomes even more pronounced. I've kept it hidden away. I tried to find other ways to cope, which chiefly meant burying my feelings and pretending everything was okay. I don't feel like grief is something that ever leaves you, and in a culture where we are so used to 'fixing ourselves' this is tough. We want an app or a therapy or a tablet that will take the pain away and recalibrate ourselves. The problem is that if you love someone and they die, then nothing will erase the loss.

I tried to escape this event but to no avail:

- I took a paracetamol overdose but I called Dad right away, so I feel like it was a cry for help. He sped me to hospital on the back of his motorbike and I promptly vomited into my crash helmet, which was even worse than having my stomach pumped.

- I ran away to live in Amsterdam, just before my 'A' level exams. I took a lot of drugs and joined a band, even though I knew at the time that this wasn't good for me. It resulted in me suffering a severe psychosis – I thought I was famous and that celebrities such as Prince and Anthony Kiedis were talking to me through their music videos. It actually was quite pleasant for me but not for my boyfriend, who had to witness me dressing up in disguise each day 'so the paparazzi won't recognise me in the supermarket again'.
- I decided to get my shit together and so came home, did my exams and then stayed in a job for eighteen years. It didn't make me happy but I did it because I was convinced I would 'stay safe' and nothing bad would happen if I didn't make any changes in my life and lived by the rules dictated by everyone else (i.e. you should work, earn money, get a mortgage if you can, etc.)

The grief became less intense, but that early trauma shaped who I am. I was lucky to survive. The fact that Janine had planned the suicide for some time was heartbreaking. I was full of anger at what she'd done to us but also felt the weight of her unhappiness pressing down on me. It was only when I became a mother myself that I caught a glimmer of the mental stress she must have been going through. I was fortunate enough that I had support and didn't suffer from severe depression. I was aware that after you have a baby it can be a dodgy time mental health-wise, so I sought treatment when I started to feel out of control.

This was chapter one of my grief journey. The lesson is this: *Don't sweep grief under the carpet and hope it goes away. It won't.*

Unfortunately, as we age, the likelihood of losing people we love becomes greater.

Chapter two of my grief journey started more recently, in March 2020. Dad died in the first week of lockdown. This time, grief was very different. His death was a shock, but he'd not been looking after himself and was an alcoholic, so it was clear that something was going to go wrong eventually. His death brought a massive amount of guilt. I was conscious I hadn't been around enough; that I'd known he wasn't well but pushed it to the back of my mind because I had a young family and was trying to earn money, 'nail it', be an excellent parent, keep fit, socialise and all the other shit we feel we have to do to justify our existence. The conversations we'd had had been quick, functional (usually about plans to see one another) and punctuated by noisy kids in the background squawking. And when I'd visited him, I'd not made an effort to engage with him. He'd hidden away in his study and I'd been too frightened to go down there because I knew he was drinking but didn't want to see if for myself (and knew he didn't want me to see it either). Like many people, I wanted to avoid unpleasant stuff, avoid his drinking, avoid his unhappiness, and he colluded in this avoidance strategy. This happens in many families – once the can of worms is cracked open, you can't get the worms back in because they've crawled up your arms and are getting into your brain via your ears where they'll take up residence if you let them.

Much of life is about learning that unpleasant emotions can't be wished away; that everyone has them to a greater or lesser degree; and they need to be felt and acknowledged and hopefully heard by someone who can take them on board without judging.

This time, I was a proper grown-up, so you'd think I'd be better equipped at dealing with loss. I'd got massive bereavement 'under my belt' and so why was this loss so much harder? I can't help thinking that losing someone you love when you're facing up to your own ageing is a tricky dynamic (remembering that it isn't a competition and everyone responds differently, but for me it threw up so many issues and challenges and still does). I felt pessimistic. I felt like this was an indication that life was only going to get worse from now on. This is a thought I still have on bad days – the negative churn – I'm getting old, there is no future, everybody dies – 'FADE OUT' by Radiohead playing on repeat until the end. I knew I would be next when it came to shuffling off this mortal coil (or I hoped I'd be next in the natural order of things). I was moving up a rung. I was the proper adult. The grown-up. I'd obviously been an adult for some time, but losing a parent made me feel like that child role had now been severely diminished. It also made the whole chapter of my step-mum and sister end abruptly – without any closure. I'd hoped to talk about it with Dad. To get some answers. In reality, there could never be any closure to what happened because there were no clear answers.

In films there is sometimes a death which brings about positive life change – the passing of a baton to the next generation – the understanding that life is fleeting and so we must appreciate each moment, but that isn't how it felt at all. Perhaps it will feel like that eventually but for now it just feels sad and empty and makes me feel tired.

There is at some point a stage of acceptance. If you look into one of the theories around grief such as that of Elizabeth Kübler-Ross and David Kessler, there are five stages: *denial, anger, bargaining, depression, acceptance*. But acceptance makes it sound as if you're okay with loss, and I'm not.

'You're behaving like a child,' someone said to me on the phone a couple of weeks after Dad's death. 'You're in your forties! You need to think about your children and grow up a bit!'

It's weird that even typing the words 'Dad's death' just then feels completely unreal. I can hear his voice in my ear, see his unsteady gait (not because of booze – he generally wobbled about a lot, even when he was young, as if his brain was taking in too much energy and his body was being dragged along behind). Yes, I'm a grown-up (well, shit, I must be at forty-seven) but grief can take you right back to the violent emotions of childhood. The vulnerability. The lack of protection. The rawness and fact that you stop regulating yourself and putting on an act. It makes you unreasonable, and that's perfectly normal. It's okay.

As a society we are seriously uncomfortable about death. Funeral parlours are strange, grey, cold, clinic-like places where death is hidden. There are catalogues to select which kind of coffin you want and then a menu of 'death services' for your delectation. Everything is sanitised. After Dad's funeral my second step-mum went to pick up his ashes. They were presented in the kind of bag that you'd get your expensive cardigan put into if you were shopping on the King's Road. It was impossible to believe that my dad – with his unruly long hair (we teased him about it as he refused to get it cut and didn't wash it often enough) and Jeremy Corbyn T-shirt (he was a big fan)… a dad who was constantly pacing about, deep in thought… who had an incredibly dry sense of humour… who had a love of very strong cheese… who secretly liked watching certain TV programmes but dismissed them as 'trash' – was inside this glossy, posh-cardigan-boutique bag. Our culture irons out the unpleasant stuff. The worms are still coming for us though. I hate to say it, but it's true.

In Max Porter's fiction book *Grief Is the Thing with Feathers*, there is a passage where the crow (playing the part of grief) arrives in the life of a man who has recently lost his wife. The crow says, 'I won't leave until you don't need me anymore.' The man replies, 'Put me down.' Then the crow says, 'Not until you say hello.' This is how I feel about grief. You have to see it, feel it and not run. There is no escape and that is overwhelming, but taking drugs or getting pissed or losing yourself in online shopping or social media are just little bursts of coming up for air. You have to go back down again, and when you do, you feel worse because you have the additional layer of guilt around your escape tactics. I don't want to take ecstasy anymore. I find a glass of rosé gives me a headache. So luckily the hedonistic route isn't open to a gal like me.

There are a few things that have helped and so I've listed them here in case you find yourself in the midst of grief (my first piece of advice would be talking about your feelings and allowing yourself to feel them in the first place).

- I listened to podcasts about grief. (There are podcasts in the Resources at the end of the book if you've recently been bereaved and want to try this.)
- I cried.
- I listened to songs that Dad loved, to feel more connection with him.
- I kept Dad's favourite jumper in a plastic bag and burrowed my head into it each evening. I will do this tonight and every night, possibly until I die. Smelling him again makes me feel better.

One of the last conversations I had with my dad was about his retirement.

'What are you going to do when you stop teaching?' I asked him on a FaceTime.

I could barely hear what he was saying because my eldest daughter had the TV on really loud and the little one was shouting in my face.

'Well, I think I might finally try and write, Nik,' he said, biting into his sausage roll (his diet got very crap towards the end). 'And then I'm going to read all of these books. I've got so many of them.' He gestured to all the shelves lining his study, which was like a cave really – a place Dad felt most comfortable in but was ultimately unhealthy as it allowed him to indulge his drinking and shut himself away too much.

I remember hanging up and feeling pleased. Writing and reading books sounded like a good retirement. Hopefully, it would also mean he'd reduce his drinking because he'd no longer be stressed at work (not that he was anyway because he loved his work as a lecturer). Dad never wrote the book. There was certainly a lot more stuff he wanted to do. The idea that death gives us a kick up the arse and makes us cry 'CARPE DIEM' is not a new one. It's a bit of a cliché – all the advice from people who have almost died or did die and basically said they wished they'd climbed Mount Kilimanjaro or learnt how to do stunts on quad bikes. There is some truth to it though. I have felt despondent most of the time but I've also felt compelled to finally write this book (which I'd been mulling over for a while) and it also gave me the impetus to make a podcast on my own, and so maybe there can be a bit of that Hollywood movie effect of death making us face up to our priorities and helping us channel our energies.

There isn't a 'right way'. I struggled because I believed that there was a process or a right way, but grief is messy. One minute you can feel fully functioning and the next you're plunged into what I can only refer to as a 'dark place'. If you think about it logically, you've lost someone that mattered and the strength of your feelings is reflected by the fact that they mattered. They're now gone from your life. This might have happened under traumatic circumstances. There is rarely the chance to say goodbye or cover all the stuff you put on the backburner under the heading 'Must Chat to Dad about This One Day'. One thing I've learned from my recent bereavement is to make sure you talk and share the things that are important and don't wait.

Grief teaches us that life (and death) is out of our control

We have apps to track our activities and count how many calories we've consumed, and apps to help us meditate, and we're used to Googling a solution to whatever we're dealing with in that moment. I've noticed that whenever something traumatic happens in my life (miscarrying a child, losing my dad) I have this knee-jerk response which is to reach for my phone and look for an answer. This is obviously absurd behaviour, but there's a sense that we feel we have control over our lives and technology builds on this idea; but when something awful happens, there's the realisation that there isn't any control at all. Losing someone we love teaches us that we may micro-manage our lives, hoping that everything goes to plan, but things will happen without warning and Google isn't going to be able to help much with that.

Dad had a ruptured aneurysm and whilst it was something that his father also had, there was no predicting that it would rupture so suddenly, or that he would go into hospital at the beginning of lockdown, or that he had a problem with alcohol which contributed to him not coming round after the surgery to save him had finished. It all happened in one afternoon. He was there, he was working and marking his students' work in his study and then by 10pm that evening he was gone. The speed of it all was unnatural to me. The following few days I texted him and even phoned him. I scrolled through endless texts and listened to his voicemails. I thought about him on that day in the hospital and how alone he'd been (we were in lockdown, not allowed to be there). As I've already flagged, the guilt was intense. Guilt that I hadn't been there; that I hadn't taken enough notice of his failing health or his increased drinking; that the last text I'd sent him had been overly formal because I was worried that I was about to lose my job. On reflection, there had been a lot of warning signs but I'd been struggling with a baby and trying to find meaningful work (being the breadwinner and working as a freelancer meant that there wasn't really any 'maternity leave). Dad had been sending me money now and then (as had my mum). I felt guilty about this too: that I was a forty-something woman being financially supported by her parents.

In essence, I spent the first three months trying to think of ways that I could have been a better daughter – more caring, more attentive, more pushy – why hadn't I driven him to a doctor and forced him to have a proper check-up when I suspected he was sick? Why had I bullied him about his excessive drinking when it was obvious that he was depressed? Why had I failed to see him in the month before he died? Why had I become more like a mother figure to him and berated him instead of offering him love and empathy? And why had we never spoken about what had happened to us: the losses and trauma we'd gone through, which had exacted a heavy toll on both of us? The guilt is still a burden: the way he died, the suddenness, the history we shared, the depression he'd obviously suffered from but never properly acknowledged and this overarching sense that I was a selfish, cruel daughter who hadn't done all I could to support and help him navigate his way through all of this.

Cariad Lloyd hosts an award-winning podcast called 'Griefcast', and in each episode she interviews a different actor/comedienne about the loss of someone they loved. One of the lovely things about it is that you learn there is no set path to grief but there are common themes and feelings. The guilt, for instance, is common. Cariad lost her dad when she was fifteen, and because she was so young perhaps, it taught her that life was a series of random events and there was not much you could depend on. If it's the first time you've lost someone and you're in your forties or fifties, then it may be your first experience of seeing life this way. Cariad elaborates on this point:

> If you come to grief quite late, it might be the first time something is completely out of your control. When I was fifteen, it gave me anxiety – it proved to me that I had no control, so it didn't matter what you read or how many times you touch wood or are grateful, people can just die.

When I lost my step-mum and sister at the same age, I spent as much time as I could trying to escape myself. I hated being alone, and still dislike it if I'm entirely honest (though writing helps as it gives me something to fill my head with when I am alone). I think my fear is that if I'm left alone for too long, I will develop a psychosis like my step-mum. This sounds absurd but I know that when I'm in the company of other people I feel safe. I chat to strangers so I can avoid the uncomfortable feelings (and maybe this is why I love podcasting too). There was no discussion of grief when I was growing up. At the funeral of my step-mum and sister, it felt like there was no acknowledgement that this was a heavy and impossible thing to manage. There was no therapy on offer, no extended period of time off school – in fact, the expectation seemed to be that life carried on as it had been before and feelings should be pushed down inside and ideally not discussed. I ran away to live in another country with an older man, and nobody saw there was a clear link between my erratic behaviour and the fact that I'd lost two beloved people. I was going to school and coming home to an empty house surrounded by traumatic memories (my father avoided coming home and spent his days and evenings at work whilst I was left on my own to prepare my own food and watch TV). And yet, I couldn't work out why I didn't feel right inside.

When Cariad lost her father, her grief manifested itself in a need to exert as much control over her world as possible – avoiding as much risk as possible in the hope that something similar wouldn't happen again:

> I didn't go down the sex and drugs and rock-and-roll route. People can die. You don't know when it's going to happen. I can't take drugs. I can't drink. Instead I was thinking that I needed to be worrying about everyone. Controlling everything. Every grief is different and unique, and the way someone dies will influence how you grieve. If it's sudden, then you're dealing with shock. If they're older, then you might be more aware, but it's not a total shock out of the blue. The way something happens will shape how you grieve.

Taking drugs is obviously not a healthy way of dealing with trauma. Some people will rely on other escapes like work, excessive exercise, drinking, online shopping and gambling. Whilst there are different ways to deal with your emotions, pushing them away isn't helpful.

There is no ready-made solution

I noticed that some of the less helpful advice was from people who were trying to tell me how to grieve, implying that there was a set process and I just had to follow the steps and would feel better. So, there were suggestions that I needed to put my dad's things away and not look at them because they were too upsetting. Or that I needed to book a holiday (as if the feelings I had wouldn't be packed away in my hand luggage and travel with me). Or that I needed to appreciate the fact I had a lovely family – and *I do appreciate my lovely family*, but it doesn't take away the fact that I miss my dad. I never really understood the 'count your blessings' mentality when people have gone through trauma.

At the moment I deal with the loss of my dad in ways which may either seem odd or entirely normal. I have a selection of photos of him, and a candle burns next to these every Friday, the anniversary of his death. I have a clean hankie of his which I keep in my pocket if I'm stressed, or under my pillow at night. I have a bag in the wardrobe containing his favourite jumper, and every night I pull it out and sink my face into it. For a moment I am in his arms again. I hear his voice. 'This is hard, Nik,' he says. 'This is hard, but you can do this.' I put the jumper away and do the normal bedtime routine with the kids. I watch TV. I seek him out in nature, thinking I can see him and imagining him walking towards me. I pretend that this is an awful joke. I also have a locket that I touch which contains a photo of the two of us. At this moment, as I write this, I need to have as many of my dad's possessions around me as possible. This is not about being in denial but more about immersing myself in the loss. I don't want to forget it and move on. I want to acknowledge what's happened and feel close to him. Is this right? Who's to say?

It's not going anywhere

I spoke to one relative and they told me that I needed to put a couple of days aside and then I could get over it more easily. Aside from this being impractical when you have a life and small children and work, it also felt prescriptive. It was the way that they'd dealt with grief, but this didn't work for me. I wanted to believe that if I did it this way, I would be quicker to heal. I also knew that missing Dad wasn't going to change if I set myself a time limit. It was going to be a constant. As I've said before, in our 'fix everything' culture it is hard to acknowledge that grief isn't fixable. There are things you can do to make yourself feel better in the moment, but it never truly leaves you. There is no app or tablet or practice that will sort it out for you (though there are tools that you can use to help and support networks you can reach out to).

Cariad feels that we need to do what we have to in order to get through it:

> Grief is a long journey and you can't fix it. It's not going away. You have to live with it in whatever way you can. You need to get the emotion out. The worst thing you can do is put it away. Yes, it's intense, and if you need to go into the woods and bash a stick against a tree, then do it. Punch a pillow. Acknowledge that it matters. It's messy. Like childbirth, you can't keep it down and be quiet. If you need to howl and scream, then do it. If you try and control it, then it takes longer. Let it be and don't judge yourself.

The idea that this is a problem that can't be fixed is a new one. It is similar to anxiety. It is always lurking and waiting to pop its ugly head up again. The most important thing is that you acknowledge the feelings and find ways to put one foot in front of other rather than wishing the thing would just go away.

'Growing around Grief'

When I first came across this concept, I clung onto the idea that there were specific stages to grief. I thought that perhaps I'd move through these emotions in a nice, tidy fashion and 'arrive' at a point where I was essentially okay with my loss. I'm not going to rubbish a theory that's been well-researched, but Cariad talks about an alternative analogy that might prove more helpful (as it doesn't make you feel like grief is a linear process – it's different for everyone).

The 'Growing around Grief' theory was created by Dr Lois Tonkin (a writer and grief counsellor) and you'll find different variations online if you do some research. She suggests drawing a circle. This circle represents you and your life and everything you're going through. You then shade in the circle and this represents your grief. So, you have a circle that is entirely shaded in and it feels like it's consuming your whole life. In essence, it impacts on everything – your sleep, eating patterns, routines – and it's impossible to think about anything else. In the past, people believed this circle got smaller. There would be change and hurt but it would perhaps get less relentless and immobilising over time. This theory also considers the idea that you can suddenly find grief overwhelming again and it never really goes away. So, for instance, Father's Day for me was rubbish, especially the first one where I saw dozens of happy dads popping up on my social media feed and felt plunged into despondency and sadness.

Choose your moments

In the first few weeks I found myself continually scrolling through photographs of Dad on my phone. I would be in the middle of feeding the kids their lunch and would listen to a voicemail he'd left me on my birthday. He sings to me and I've played it so many times – pausing and rewinding it so that I can parrot it back verbatim. I found the fact that I had so much digital information bewildering – intense pain was at my fingertips and I could dip into it at any time. I became obsessed with the idea that my dad was now somewhere in our house, as he used to share his location and it now looked as if his phone was hovering over our address (it was my phone, of course, as his had been switched off). I also spent an inordinate amount of time holding my finger down on LIVE photos I'd taken on my phone so I could hear snippets of what he was saying (to see if they were significant things, which of course they weren't). The issue is that when we are addicted to our phone, there's a temptation to look through old photos, and that can suddenly send you right back into the centre of a grief whirlpool. I still find myself doing these deep, immersive grief dives at different times (photos/emails/texts) but I try and be a bit more thoughtful about whether it's a good time, whether I need it, whether it might be better to be kind to myself and leave that dive to another time.

The stories live on after the person has gone

It sounds like a cliché but nobody can take away the memories you have. Dad liked to eat strong cheese. He always liked to smoke a pipe and then moved onto a vape. He once sat on a tray and slid on his bum down a sand dune in New Zealand. He liked beer gardens. And dogs. He used to call me 'Pumpkin'. He was obsessed with pigs. He drew a pig smoking a pipe on every letter he sent me. He was a great writer. He played piano and people went silent when he played. He refused to cut his hair. He liked to hug. When I was small, his arms would envelop me and he'd make this noise like a grizzly bear and I could feel his chest vibrating against mine and I was safe. He made me sit up late completing maths and science projects. He once conducted an orchestra in the garden. He was a Doctor of Philosophy. He loved liquorice. The saltier the better. He worked in the anti-apartheid movement in South Africa and was a fundraiser for a division of the ANC. He was nocturnal. He worked at night. He lost his wife and child. He loved to travel. And these are just a few of the things I know about him, and nobody can ever take them away.

Losing a parent is discombobulating, and grief isn't a competition

Another thing I noticed about grief is that there can be a subtle tendency (sometimes not so subtle) for people to be competitive about it. Or maybe it's supposed to offer some kind of reassurance. So, they may tell you that they lost someone who was closer to them/under more traumatic circumstances, etc. This is true with many emotional journeys, but it's not a competition. You can feel intense grief whatever your relationship was with that person. And it is no less traumatic to the person if they miscarried a baby or lost a person they loved. The flavour may be different, but it's interesting that many seem to assume that losing babies through miscarrying them isn't so bad because they weren't born yet so didn't quite have their own identities. Or there may be others who try and point out a 'bright side' and say things like 'Well, he had a good innings' or 'He was depressed and is at peace now'. The vast majority of this stuff is just people struggling to come up with the 'right thing' to say when there isn't anything that sounds right. The only right thing is to acknowledge that losing someone is awful and that you're there to support. If you've experienced grief yourself, you'll know that none of these comments make any difference, because you exist inside a bubble of grief and it's impenetrable, and whilst you appreciate people reaching out and trying to penetrate that bubble, it's not going to have a significant impact (I don't want to discourage people from supporting their friends or family who are grieving, but in the initial stages you could be speaking a foreign language and they possibly wouldn't notice). When I meet people who have suffered loss, I feel there is a flicker of recognition in our eyes. There is a sense that they've been through something heavy and are carrying it with them.

One friend told me she'd just lost her aunt and I immediately felt competitive myself – like losing an aunt wasn't as important as losing your dad. It doesn't matter WHO has died – everyone will experience pain, feel weird, sad and vulnerable. We shouldn't get competitive. This is true of all miserable experiences – there isn't a 'winner' when it comes to who feels worse. For me, losing a parent made me feel vulnerable and as if I'd lost a significant part of 'what makes me me'. Cariad Lloyd also had similar emotions, despite being a child when she lost her dad:

> Whatever age you are, it's going to affect you. Your parents do provide an essence of your identity. And when that goes, the ground shakes under your feet. Grieving is about rebuilding that ground and that takes a long time.

And this is the thing about ageing, it's ultimately facing up to our own mortality. Once Dad died, I realised that I was moving up a tier and getting closer to meeting my Maker too. I also realised I had to reassess where my life was going and make some changes. So whilst it's broken my heart and I won't ever 'recover' from it (you don't), I feel that one positive is that it's making me think about the next phase of my life and I'm also visualising Dad and what he'd say if he could see me writing this right now. And he is watching. I feel that now. And he's saying, 'Nik,' (he always called me this – nobody else calls me this anymore, which makes me sad too) 'you're doing a great job. Keep going. Keep it up.'

And that offers me solace of sorts.

What if we got it all wrong and a busy distracted life wasn't the way forward?

Sometimes I try and visualise that moment at the pearly gates. God is standing there, but she's female so a Goddess, and has this yellow aura around her body and she floats in the air and doesn't really have a face or a body – like a transparent omelette.

'So why should we let you into heaven?' she says, this holy, yellow blob of goodness. 'Did you live a good life full of purpose?'

In my visualisation, I'm feeling slightly shell-shocked because I've fallen out of my stand-up bath (despite the adverts saying this is impossible) and suffered a catastrophic head wound, and I'm thinking about how unfortunate it is to be discovered naked by the ambulance crew, and how I wish I'd at least been able to grab a towel. And now here I am standing in front of the Goddess (I never believed in heaven but I am relieved there is one).

'Well I worked hard and I bought a house and I was a feminist, so I always had my own money and didn't rely on anyone else for cash. I also tried to use Ecover toilet cleaner whenever I could but found the ecological washing powder not so great. It left stains – especially on the kids' clothes, so I'm afraid I used Persil and now and then I'd resort to bleach when the toilet was really dirty – you know how it is with small kids? I also recycled and never littered, and I did a couple of runs for charity – not the Marathon, I wasn't fit enough to do the Marathon and find running for that long boring unless there's a good podcast, but then my knees started playing up… but I tried to help people too.'

'But what did you do with your life? What was your purpose?' the Goddess blob booms back at me (with the voice of a very authoritarian man – not what I expected from this yellow blob at all).

'Well I was a mum. I had a career. I worked really hard – probably too hard, actually – and I was an okay mum but not one of those that throws her entire life into it, so I didn't bake or do loads of craft and I sometimes resented the kids and found them annoying and wished I could lie down and just watch TV like I did before they were born.'

'You're still not telling me what you actually did with your life? What was your purpose?'

'To be happy sometimes?'

'That's not a purpose!'

'To be productive?'

'That's not your purpose.'

'I loved my friends and my family and my partner.'

'No sorry that's not enough.'

'I had a career?'

'No.'

'I had a lot of followers on Instagram before they bought out that new platform BIG BOOM and everyone wore virtual reality helmets and Instagram went down the pan?'

'No.'

Then I'll be stuck and not know what to say.

'So, you never actually thought about your purpose?' the Goddess says. 'You never thought about how you wanted to live or whether you were living the right way?'

'Do you mean I should have gone to church? I did go a bit and I believed in heaven, or at least I wanted to, but I never got round to thinking about big stuff. I guess I was hedging my bets a little.'

'What did you do instead?'

'I always had a lot of stuff to be getting on with – you know, the career, the kids, social media, watching loads of Netflix, exercise, tidying the house, replying to all those messages on my phone, buying presents for kids' parties. I mean, even later on I thought things would slow down but the social media just got more intense and I was trying to update my status and tell people about my new stand-up bath. (That's actually how I fell out. I was trying to reply to a message on that new platform BIG BOOM and shouldn't have been wearing my virtual reality helmet and I think it must have come off and my head crashed onto the bathroom floor.)'

The Goddess would stare at me then. Her expression is a mix of contempt and pity.

'I have been watching you all your life. I have been watching you and you have spent your entire life being distracted. There have been the odd few moments here and there where you've been present – like when you were giving birth, for instance.'

'Yes, I definitely was present then.'

'And when you lost your dad.'

'Yes, that's true.'

'And during the coronavirus crisis.'

'Yes, yes. I was definitely present and thought about my purpose then.'

'But the rest of the time you were just dashing about and not thinking. You were buying into an idea that everyone bought into – this idea that the busier you are, the more money you have, the more productive a person you are, the better life you have.'

I pause and just stare – realising that, yes, my life – a lot of my life – has been lived on autopilot.

'And you were lying when you said you used Ecover. I saw you bleach the toilet many times.'

And I try and contradict her but realise that, yes, this is true too. I haven't even helped the planet in my own small way. I've instead contributed to the pollution and global warming and been selfish because I didn't want giant skid marks in the toilet.

'Can I come into heaven?' I ask sheepishly.

'What have you learnt?'

'I've learnt that I probably focused too much on comparing myself to others and trying to have material success.'

'You're halfway there, but you still have a lot to learn. You can come in but you will need to prove you can appreciate the important things and stop focusing on the stuff that really doesn't matter. For a start, we need to wean you off BIG BOOM.'

'I promise,' I reply.

And the Goddess reaches her arms out to me and I'm absorbed into her yellow light and I float and close my eyes but I have one final question to ask before I became part of her being – ready to welcome more people into heaven but no longer owning a body of my own.

'Did the ambulance man see my bum when I fell out the bath?'

And the Goddess smiles (or I feel her smile like a warm rain massaging my temples).

'Yes, he did, but he didn't care because at the end of the day your butt, your old lady butt, really doesn't matter, does it?'

Then, just before I disappear or my body disappears, I feel a presence and it's my dad, his arms on my shoulders, because he's been waiting for many years, just as he said he would in my dream, and I say something like 'I knew there was more, that I needed to change, and I tried and sometimes I did, but ultimately I have a long way to go.' He doesn't contradict me, even though he liked arguing when we were both alive, and we embrace this puzzling idea of heaven – a heaven where you get second chances.

I'll be ready.

CHAPTER TWELVE

The Modern Addiction to Busy-ness, and Why We Need to CHILL THE F%*K OUT

Have you ever noticed that whenever you talk to someone or read a celebrity interview or see people on Instagram, they're always talking up how busy they are? The notion that we don't have any time, that we are constantly filling up every single second with productive activities, that we are stressed and our eyeballs are bulging because we're so rushed off our feet. Hasn't that felt like the modern malaise for quite some time now?

Let's compare and contrast the life of a woman in her forties in the 1990s with a woman in her forties in the current times:

1990s woman
- Get up.
- Get kids ready for childcare/school.
- Commute to work (read paper/stare out window/at weird man winking at me).
- Work in office at computer – send emails and expect responses following day, send some faxes.
- Have lunch – maybe at desk (let's face it, this has been going on since office life began and is a good way of demonstrating to your boss that you're super-busy).
- Send more emails and write stuff.

- Commute home (more staring, maybe some reading if have remembered book, maybe even a nap if can sit down).
- Pick up kids.
- Make dinner (usually throw frozen stuff into the fryer – well this was my childhood sometimes).
- Kids watch TV.
- Bathtime.
- Bedtime.
- Watch TV, read a book, go to bed.

2020 woman

- Get up at 5am (based on theory that you should be awake for an hour before everyone else so you can be productive and do stuff).
- Meditate.
- Check social media.
- Send emails.
- Get kids up, suddenly realise there is a special 'dress-up day' at school and try and make a World Book Day outfit from a duster and a pair of PE shorts.
- Apply make-up (after cleansing, toning and applying serum, SPF and CC cream) and hair serum, exfoliate body, apply fake tan, get dressed.
- Run to school, checking emails (already have thirty+ that require responses IMMEDIATELY).
- Get to tube/bus and reply to mails, listen to a podcast, watch an episode of something, check social media, reply to pissed-off messages from mums on WhatsApp who have realised they have missed World Book Day or smug bastards who have spent three weeks making a Hobbit outfit from Shredded Wheat boxes and string.
- Run to office, stare at phone, type up replies, neck coffee.

- First meeting commences. Run out and get coffee.
- Second meeting (it's only 11am).
- Back at desk. Update social media, reply to twenty emails, log into online childcare portal to see if youngest kid is okay and has eaten something. Work for an hour.
- Lunch (eaten at desk but probably tastier than that of a 90s woman who had to eat white bread sandwich with cheese and Marmite brought in from home).
- Back at desk but then another meeting.
- Check emails during meeting but then realise this is rude so take notes instead.
- End of meeting. Back at desk. Do some work, check social media, get up and have a coffee, do more work, order new school uniform socks, book tickets for school play but can't access school website, go into another meeting, text a friend who is having a bad time.
- Try and write some ideas for podcast/book/new life on tube, then start listening to a podcast but then start watching a Netflix series, then panic as realise have forgotten to reply to important email. Get off tube, go above ground, send email, get back on.
- Pick kids up.
- Cook dinner (pasta but with vegetables. Ideally, and no fried shit).
- Bedtime (which takes a long time as am no longer allowed to shout 'GO TO BED AND SHUT UP OR A MONSTER WILL EAT YOU UP' or whatever it was 1990s parents shouted up the stairs (they weren't as worried and uptight about their parenting as us, you see).
- Watch TV whilst scrolling through social media, liking photos that make us anxious, checking work emails and WhatsApp and then watching TV.

- Go to bed but toss and turn as brain whirrs on and on with a million bits of trivial and not-so-trivial stuff to do tomorrow.

A few differences between the 1990s woman and the modern-day one

- For a start, the 1990s woman stared a lot more.
- She didn't have a little machine that gave her stuff to do and look at all the time and so would spend more time thinking, and maybe fantasising about Pierce Brosnan or her co-worker, or devising really interesting creative ideas or just counting the number of stripes on the seat pattern opposite her.
- If she forgot World Book Day, then nobody gave a shit (and there was no WhatsApp to make her feel judged/shit).
- The expectations around work were different. It was acceptable to go home and not have to do more paid work.
- Nobody cared what her kids had for dinner, as long as they were fed.
- There were not acres of content to consume, sending her into a panic of paralysis (i.e. how do you choose between a podcast/audio book/Netflix series/reading/social media when it's all at your fingertips every minute of the day?).
- There was no social media, so she might compare herself to a co-worker or a friend *but* she was not comparing herself to thousands of strangers.
- There was an understanding that being productive 24/7 was perhaps only something that people did when they were going through a manic episode and were about to crash and burn and possibly end up in a psychiatric hospital for six months.

IT'S JUST TOO TIRING. By the time we get to our forties and mid-forties the cult of busy-ness really does kick us right up the proverbial butt. When you're in your twenties it's kind of okay to be busy, because you have bags of energy and you only really have yourself to care for – you can work late, or just keep on working and carry on, and be okay (though you will get burn-out eventually). Some of us can even carry on with the filling-every-moment-of-every-day-with-stuff in our thirties (though we may start to suffer health problems).

Then once you get past forty, if you continue trying to do everything and be everything and achieve everything and never give your brain ten minutes to stare or absorb the world around you, you notice strange things happening:

- You start getting heart palpitations.
- You fantasise about strangling tourists who walk too slowly in front of you.
- You hop from foot to foot whilst waiting for your coffee order.
- You swear, but not in a fun way – instead in a way that makes people raise their eyebrows and feel afraid.
- You talk to yourself in public.
- Your bottom lip quivers when someone asks you how you are.
- You reveal very personal information to someone you don't know (i.e. the lady in the post office).
- You are livid.
- You wake up in the mornings and cannot get out of bed – you have to crawl first and then stand up.

Eventually (or this is what happened to me) you start to question why this busy-vibe thing has taken over. Where is the reward at the end of the day? Is there a medal for being the busiest person in the universe? When do we get the medal? If not, why bother?

Out of the survey I did, 76 per cent of women said they were feeling more overwhelmed as they grew older, and 72 per cent felt they were saddled with all the household admin and housework. Here are some typical examples of comments they shared:

> The life admin is ever growing and the night worries are getting stronger.

> It's impossible to keep on top of everything, I find. With long working hours, looking after kids and then keeping the home tidy and organised, I feel overwhelmed.

> I want to stop working so home life becomes more manageable. At the moment it feels like I'm not doing anything properly.

The truth is, our lives have changed since the 1990s. Nowadays we are often working in a similar pattern to men, with long hours, no clear divide between work and family and then doing all the domestic organisation – keeping on top of the house cleaning and tidying through to ensuring the kids' stuff is all in order (the playdates/non uniform 'fun' days/checking homework/birthday parties/buying presents/all that shizzle). Lockdown has actually amplified our workloads, with women taking on more of the domestic chores and child-related admin. This was discussed in an article in *The Guardian* – the fact that women have had to bear the brunt of the mental load since the lockdown started. Rachel Sklar, a single mum and gender advocate, put it thus:

> There's the Covid-19 mental load: Are we ready? What do we need? Fear of what's going to happen. And then there is the mental load of the single parent in a one-income household after terrifying market drops and business grinding to a standstill.

For a single parent there isn't the option of asking their partner to help out. (Interestingly, women with a partner also seem to do all the small stuff, whether there's a pandemic on or not.) It was interesting that during lockdown all the WhatsApp conversations tended to be around the kids and the school work that was being set each week – whether it was enough, whether it was being commented on by the teachers, whether the kids needed to be doing more or less. All the responsibility had landed on the mums in terms of setting tasks up, uploading them onto the platforms, and checking to see each day if there was more. This sort of stuff, the 'nitty gritty shitty' of family life, is the reason why so many women are grumpy and tired and pissed off.

Sometimes, however, women can be their own worst enemies. I've often been guilty of doing stuff and feeling resentful about it but never actually telling my other half that I want him to help. This is the first lesson of overwhelm: ASK FOR HELP and stop being a bloody martyr.

These kind of conversations between women are very common. They have been going on for centuries but today they are even more tedious because women are supposed to have more equal roles with men.

'God, I had to get up in the night again with the baby and he was just snoring his head off and wouldn't wake up.'

'I know. I had to order all the uniform for the start of term and he didn't even notice they'd grown out of it already.'

'I hate it when he leaves the empty loo roll just hanging in the loo-roll holder.'

'The bath toys are just all over the floor when I go in and there's been no effort to pick them up and put them away.'

Sound familiar?

With small kids there is often that sense that we walk around the house picking things up and putting them down somewhere else. It also feels like we are the only ones in the house that have got a system in terms of where these things go. My partner is very hands on with the children but nonetheless it is me who takes a bag stuffed with wet wipes, nappies, drinks, snacks, change of clothes, coat, muslins, sun cream, and a sun hat if we're going out. He picks up his car keys and his sunglasses and goes. It is all on my shoulders to think about these things and I sometimes feel like it prevents me from being a genius or just feeling less drained every day (or even just doing more staring, which is what I feel I need to do).

The biggest lesson I have learnt is to SAY SOMETHING to my partner and stop feeling that he'll pick up on my grumpy mood through keen observation. When I do say something, more often than not he is willing to take more on but has assumed that I was happy doing it. The other thing I've learnt is you have to relinquish control. You cannot ask someone to do something and then get obsessed with the idea that they must do it exactly how you would do it. Yes, if they hang the loo roll over the bannister, that's fundamentally not right; but if they decide to buy a present for a kids' party and it's not the thing that you would have bought, then don't have a fit about it. I've noticed with friends that there is often the long whinge about how their partners aren't helping with certain stuff; but when their partners do stuff, then they whinge about how they've not done the stuff to a certain standard (I'm guilty of this too but am working on it). In her brilliant book about relationships after having children, *How Not to Hate Your Husband after Kids*, author Jancee Dunn says:

> For all my complaints that I want Tom to be more involved, he counters that I jump in and micromanage when he does... I would hurriedly check after he had changed a loaded diaper for what is commonly known in my circle of mums as 'butt rust'. I must admit that when it comes to kid-related tasks I feel I do a more conscientious job.

This idea that we do it better, so we must do it, is not a good one and perpetuates the grumpy woman syndrome. This is especially true when we get older and have those peri-menopausal/menopausal hormones pumping around and feel more tired because we're older and have more of a need to just sit down and stare at a wall like our 1990s counterparts did back in the day.

We live in a society where our understanding of what success looks like has changed. In the cave woman days, success would have been getting to the end of the day without being eaten by a bear. For the Tudor woman, it would have been not succumbing to plague or smallpox before she hit twenty-five. For the 90s woman, it would have been holding down a job (not necessarily an interesting job, just being employed) and bringing up kids. For us today, it's whether we have an interesting/fulfilling/brag-worthy job, have raised bright, well-rounded children, written a book, hosted a podcast, got a kitchen extension, run 10k that day, had sex, absorbed at least 2–3 examples of content that everyone is talking about so can chat about it in an informed way, posted something witty but not too smug on social media, kept up to speed with all the messages that fly into our weary, blurry eyes like flies hitting a car window screen at high speed, cleaned the toilet, wormed the cat, maintained our friendships, cooked, cleaned and tidied. (It actually makes the being eaten by a bear days sound okay.)

I am addicted to my smartphone. I carry it with me wherever I am. Increasingly, I look at it whilst I'm doing other stuff (like watching TV or reading a magazine or having a conversation). I can't tear my eyes away from it most of the time. I know that my relationship with my phone isn't healthy and I also know what my life was like before they were invented, because I lived most of my life without one. (I used to laugh when I saw people in the street with mobile phones and thought they were giant wankers, but I am now a giant wanker just like everyone else.)

I spoke to psychotherapist and author of *The Phone Addiction Workbook*, Hilda Burke, who also specialises in counselling clients about overwhelm and their addiction to their phones. First off, I asked her whether women are putting too much pressure on themselves these days and whether we're often our own worst enemies. Hilda agreed:

> If there is a track record of excelling and always doing well, then they can bring this into their child rearing too and get frustrated that they're not achieving all their goals at home. There is still a sense that it's never enough – in terms of what they're achieving and what their children are achieving. There are also social and cultural expectations.

How to avoid feeling overwhelmed all the damn time

Set your own expectations rather than live up to those of others

We were raised to believe that we could have it all and, by extension, do it all too. However, it's interesting that during the coronavirus lockdown a lot of women have felt that the level of 'managing everything' is simply too much. It's important that we take a step back and think about WHO we are trying to impress. Are we expecting teachers to congratulate us on how well we have managed? Or that partners will buy us dinner when it's all over because we shouldered all the emotional turmoil? Instead, it's a case of thinking what you feel is important versus looking for external validation.

Your brain can only take in so much stuff, so just stop taking in so much stuff all the time, okay?

Earlier this year I was living a lifestyle that wasn't sustainable. I was trying to work, bring up kids and launch my side hustle bollocks (i.e. writing/podcasting), and was feeling permanently tired and fed up. Phones and technology also contribute to this – they drive that sense of always being 'on' and always having to check things. You have to fill up every moment of time. So, I'll be having a bath and at the same time I'll be trying to browse my podcast library and look at audio books, and then there's a magazine that's landed through the door. I'm unable to just do nothing and sit in the bath and stare without feeling guilty. Hilda talks about this in more detail:

> I have a client who, after many years of working through her lunch, started taking a lunch break after she acknowledged that she needed some time to down tools halfway through her day. However, what I discovered was that she used her break to listen to podcasts which were all related to work and so her mind was never switching off. Educational and 'self-improvement' podcasts or Ted Talks can be particularly insidious when what we actually need [people] to be doing is switching off and not consuming new concepts. We need time to not be taking in new ideas.

We are never truly 'off' anymore

Hilda talks more about the culture we live in now:

> The drive to be productive can be very corrosive. We need time to do nothing in order to focus well when we actually need to do work. Another client of mine admitted that they were never fully 'on' or fully 'off' – so checking email, doing social media, watching YouTube during work hours meant that they felt they needed to work weekends in order to catch up on their job. Before all this tech, we had less distractions – there was a sense of a day's work and then going home; the work–life boundaries were more clearly defined.

*Smartphones are horrible, demanding
little monkey bastards*

I've found it nigh on impossible to stop checking my phone. It's become so bad. I have read accounts of how people during the coronavirus lockdown have become all in touch with their true selves and made banana bread and become more authentic. Yes, in some ways I've done that (I've certainly thought more about what I want from life), but the truth is I've mainly been doing the following:

This is a typical interaction with my phone. I might have picked it up just to have a little peek whilst preparing dinner for example…

Me: [Peers at Instagram story post.] *How the fuck did they manage to get subtitles on their Instagram story?* [Looks in App store for half an hour and buys an app, but then realises it charges a subscription fee of £15.99 a week.]

Me: *This gal has even got an animation thing for her podcast and has put some jazzy giphys in there. How do I do that? Oh, does anyone even look at this stuff? Well I'm looking at it so I guess they do right?* [Goes back into App store and tries to find the right app and eventually lands on something but it causes phone to break immediately. Eventually gets it working again.]

Me: *Shit. Everyone is so much better at me at Instagram. They're all jazzy and technical and doing all these subtitles and funny animations. I'm old.* [Starts to look at images of women who are younger, have smoother skin, less cellulite – some of whom are going on about how they love their non-airbrushed bodies, even though it's obvious that they don't need any airbrushing in the first place.]

Me: *I wonder… If I upload more photos of myself with cellulite, will I get more followers? Hang on, I've got a direct message.*

[Checks message.] *Oh, it's a military man in Kansas called George and he's 74. Why do these men keep messaging me? What's going on? Why can't it be Cillian Murphy?* [Googles 'Does Cillian Murphy have a girlfriend?' Then 'Real age of Cillian Murphy's girlfriend?' Then hovers on an image of said girlfriend and enlarges it to check out whether she has frown lines or not. Then tries to get app working so can put subtitles on story which was original focus anyway.] *Oh, there's nobody going to watch my stories anyway. My chin is sagging. I need to hold the phone up higher, but then it's obvious. I wonder... If I tie it up with an elastic band will it make a difference?* [Goes off in search of elastic band.]

By now, forty minutes have passed. This could have been forty minutes spent doing some writing or phoning a friend, or even just doing absolutely nothing, but instead I've wasted time just dicking about on Instagram and now feel demotivated and tired.

How to have a healthier relationship with your phone

One of the biggest things is trying to develop a more aware and mindful relationship with your phone. This means not letting it control you and take over your life. Remember that the monkey is an exciting monkey and has lots of fun things to show you. Is it any wonder that phones have become more interesting than our partners? If you want to be able to access bright colours, lovely things, news, the outside world, friends, and all sorts of other stuff, then your phone is always going to be more attractive than your other half. (I've not really touched on the impact they have on our relationships, but it's not unusual now to see couples in restaurants, sitting in silence and browsing online instead. This always make me yearn for the days when couples used to just sit in silence, staring at one another instead – those good old days!)

Hilda Burke has the following tips on how to develop a healthier relationship with your phone. These are all things that will help you feel more in control and wean you off the unhealthy feeling of always being 'ON' (with the knock-on effect of feeling overwhelmed).

- Switch off alerts and notifications, so you don't feel tempted to keep checking to see what you're missing.
- Remove social media apps from your phone – and access them on your laptop – you can do this for a week or try it for a couple of days. This will help you understand how much time you're spending mindlessly scrolling and also check how you feel.
- Switch your phone off – this is radical but if you feel like you really need a break but can't avoid temptation, try this for a short period of time and note how much angst you feel. For starters, maybe leave it at home when you go for a walk.
- Once you've got used to being apart from your phone for longer periods, have a whole day off. Turn off the data so you can call people but there's no email or messages –this can obviously only be done if you're not working and aren't expecting any important stuff that day.
- Avoid checking your phone in the morning (so have an hour without it first thing) and do this at night too (so no phone for an hour before bed – don't stimulate yourself too much and have boundaries).

Social media – check yourself

With social media it's important to notice how it makes you feel. Sometimes it can be great (e.g. a lovely message from a friend) but at other times it can leave you feeling crap. For me, it often contributes to a sense that I'm not doing enough or not parenting well enough (e.g. if I find out other parents have been doing craft or have made a lovely quinoa salad with kale and pine nuts, but we've had a shit day at home with arguments and conflict and I've only managed to make baked beans on toast). Then there's the whole way you look as you get older. You see other people on social media looking amazing and having a great social life and it makes you feel glum. I tend to look at Instagram first thing and feel drained by it. Hilda says we need to be more mindful:

> A morning routine is particularly crucial – it sets the tone for the day so it is really important. Often clients will say that their day started badly when they got a stressful message from their boss or saw their ex on social media. How can we be more conscious about that and have more agency? It's worth reflecting on who you follow and what you're inviting into your life.

Avoid looking at your competition when you're working on something

For me, this is other writers. I tend to look at their feeds, and I'm like, 'FUCK! Their book is in the bestseller list and there's no point in writing. I might as well just give up.' Hilda also had this experience:

> Starting any creative process, you need to incubate your project. When I started writing my book, I made a decision not to check what other writers had published on the same topic I was focusing on. It wouldn't have been helpful to discover that there was a Harvard professor who had written a bestselling tome on the same subject. It's important to give your own voice space to develop and grow, and comparison with others' efforts is incredibly unhelpful.

Doing nothing is a life skill

Lying down and looking at the sky for an hour and allowing that void is important – an empty vessel. You can take in a lot after you've emptied your mind, but when it's full to the brim, you can't. Doing nothing is important for our brain and wellbeing. It's like that with physical exercise, too – personal trainers advise having two days a week when you do very little exercise. Think about this in terms of your brain. You need 20 per cent downtime, so what would that look like? It would mean two hours a day not reading or watching TV. That's hard because our culture and society are all about what you have read and what you have done. A lot of us get hooked on that.

*Be more aware of some of the stuff
you read in the media*

Beware of absorbing too much information around the routines of super-successful people. As I've mentioned before, whenever I pick up a magazine there's always a profile of a super-successful woman and her average routine. I've flagged up why these routines are shit (they make us feel inadequate), but there's also another reason why they're not helpful. When we read these things, we don't realise that we're celebrating success in very narrow terms (i.e. success = being rich). The women being celebrated are often successful in one area of their lives. Of course, it's impressive, but we don't find out what the rest of their life looks like. We're given a sense that if we just work harder, we can achieve it too. If you combine this tension with a sense of 'time running out', it can be the kind of cocktail to push you over the edge into crazy, peri-menopausal breakdown. Let's take the example of Victoria Beckham. I have nothing against her, but she's obviously got a team behind her doing childcare, admin, cleaning, diaries, facials (I bet she has a 'chief chin hair plucker' on the payroll too). Let's just be honest and say, 'YES, WELL DONE, BUT I COULD LAUNCH MY OWN LIPSTICK BRAND, TOO, IF I HAD THE STAFF. GIVE ME THE FUCKING STAFF AND I'LL SHOW YOU WHAT

I CAN DO!' Hilda talks more about this dynamic of only seeing a glimpse of female success and how it adds to the mental load:

> We value successful career people and we don't look at their family relationships, their friendships or how content they are. We may focus on the fact that they run a company, are at the pinnacle of their career and are successful. But that's just one external aspect of their lives. We're not considering their lives 'in the round' – we don't know whether they might be addicted to their work and feel worthless without it.

If you can get some help around the house, then why not do it?

I sometimes feel like women are embarrassed to come forward and say they pay people to help them. They might whisper 'I got a cleaner' and then give you a look as if you're going to judge them. I can't afford a cleaner but, BELIEVE ME, if I could then I would definitely have one. I don't enjoy scrubbing the toilet or trying to get dried toothpaste out of the sink. I don't like hoovering up hardened food on the carpet. Instead of spending time doing these chores, I could enjoy either DOING NOTHING, as Hilda advises, or launching my own lipstick range and making millions. I am tired of reading profiles of celebrity women where the interviewer celebrates just how busy they are and how they're ultimately nailing it.

> **Interviewer:** I just can't believe how much you've accomplished. You have a beautiful home, four children, your own fashion line, a successful charity venture, and now you've just launched your own range of skin serums for poodles. How do you fit it all in?

Celebrity: [Throwing head back and laughing.] I just have a lot of determination. I enjoy being busy. I think it's great to have a lot on – I love the challenge of it.

NO, NO, NO. SHUT UP, SHUT UP, SHUT UP. This is really what we need to hear instead:

Interviewer: I just can't believe how much you've accomplished. You have a beautiful home, four children, your own fashion line, a successful charity venture, and now you've just launched your own range of skin serums for poodles. How do you fit it all in?

Celebrity: Listen up, friend. I have a lot of help. I have a nanny who looks after my kids so I can go to the gym. I have a cleaner who tidies the entire house each day and does the washing. I even have a cook who makes all the meals. I'd be fucking exhausted if I ran a business and did all the other stuff. Let's stop peddling the idea that it's realistic to have it all. Let's get real.

A short aside on how I really feel about Instagram

Sometimes we can start believing that Instagram is our life rather than a platform on which to share stuff. I've seen some women on there and it feels like their every waking moment is documented for social media. When it's your business and the main source of income, then it's one thing (there's still a need to live life away from it though), but when it's living for Instagram, performing for it, constantly thinking about how to capture a moment to share with your followers, then it can be a massive drain.

I have at times had an unhealthy relationship with social media and this manifests itself in a couple of ways:

1. I sometimes lose sight of the fact that writing posts and updates and stories on Instagram is not my reason for living.
2. I also feel like I have this dual lens and I'm seeing life through the lens of Instagram and thinking, 'Oh this would be a good picture to put up' or 'I love this stupid animation and need to share it right away'.

I realise that this is unhealthy. I've had a difficult relationship with social media. When I was going through trouble having kids, I hated it as everyone was sharing photos of their newborn babies, and then those cards that display how many weeks old they are accompanied by gorgeous photos of the baby, etc. It was torture. Then when I was finally a mum finally and got involved in editing the Selfish Mother blog, I found that Instagram was a great tool. I could drop a message to someone and usually they'd reply quickly. And if I was working on an article or a blog, there was this whole network of helpful people. I made some excellent friends and found that there was this strange intimacy – we went straight to the meat of the stuff that mattered rather than talking all around the edges. I found support and love, and often it was great. I also found that it could make me feel incredibly needy. If I looked at it at the wrong time, I would go into a negative spiral, wondering why more people didn't like my posts or why someone else was so much better than me at filming themselves talking. I generally have found that I feel better, safer and more robust when I'm not spending long periods of time on Instagram (I use the Forest app to stop myself picking my phone up if I'm writing or simply feel frazzled by it all).

Instagram can literally become more like your life than your actual life (so you spend more time thinking about how to post something interesting about your life on Instagram versus actually having an interesting life). Then there's the comparison thing. There was a time a couple of years ago when I was clearly nowhere near where I wanted to be in my life, and I found the endless updates of women who were nailing it and bossing it and all that shizz were exhausting (just like the newborns had been). I also didn't enjoy the events and panels (which have died down now because of the pandemic) because they felt so artificial and weird. It was like speed dating but worse. I remember going to a book launch with my friend Amy (who wasn't on Instagram at that time). The conversation went like this:

'Why is everyone looking over one another's' shoulders?' she asked me.

It was a cramped basement in Soho, and it was true – every person in there was scanning the room to see who'd just come in, and whether that person had a lot of followers and would therefore be an ideal candidate to get a selfie with.

'The problem,' I said, 'is that there's always someone more influential than you and that feeling sucks.'

'Shit, are you kidding? How old are these women?' Amy replied in horror. 'I mean the free stuff is obviously cool and I love these mini-champagne bottles, but we're in our forties! This feels like school. Even worse than school.'

'Hang on, see that woman there?' I replied, ignoring her. 'That's the biggest fashion influencer on the planet. She has literally gazillions of people following her.'

'I don't recognise her,' Amy said, taking another glug of her free champagne.

'You're not on Instagram, you fool,' I replied.

'Look at that woman over there. She's practically shoving her phone in that poor person's face!'

'She's trying to get a selfie. If she gets a selfie, then she might get more followers.'

'Jeez. I'm not sure I can hang around here much longer. Can't we just go to Pizza Express and get a four-cheese pizza?'

'I need to network a bit,' I said. 'I'll be back in five.'

I walked about the room. A couple of the heavyweight influencers blanked me (there was this implicit understanding that you approached them and paid homage but never the other way round). If I did find myself being chatted up by one of them, it was usually because of my connection to another influencer (who was actually really nice and down-to-earth and completely normal). Anyway, we left the event and had a pizza and all was well.

I have never sat smack bang in the middle of the Instagram world. I will be completely honest and also say that a couple of years back I bought some followers because I thought it would help me make it as a writer. I thought I'd be more likely to get a book deal and I could finally follow my dreams. I suspect a lot of people do this but don't talk about it. It didn't have any impact on my publishing career. I still had to get a deal the way everyone else does. I managed to get an agent and then my agent sent my manuscript off to lots of people. Most of the influencers I've met have been okay people. Some of them have been absolute horrors, but that's true of any random group of women you meet in a room. There is, however, a definite pecking order and if you're prone to insecurity, then it's not an entirely healthy dynamic. I often felt like I wasn't cool enough, and when I opened up to others about this fear, they oftentimes admitted they felt the same. I was once invited to lunch at a hotel (I rarely get any freebies – probably because I'm too old and not attractive enough – but this time the lunch was free). The lunch was for a TV broadcaster. There'd obviously been a mistake as the other attendees were all in their twenties and YOUTUBE stars. They'd set tripods up next to their plates and recorded videos of the lunch and didn't speak to one another at all. I stared at my plate and took a couple of photos of my food.

'I've just been asked to do a video for the Bulgarian Tourist Board,' the girl next to me said. 'I'm getting an all expenses trip and then I just have to make a couple of videos. Top hotel the whole lot.'

She was very pretty and had a lot of make up on. I worked out I could possibly be her mum and thought that perhaps the PR woman on the other side of me thought this was who I was – otherwise, what was I doing here? The guy on the far side of the table was glued to his phone and wasn't eating a morsel of his delicious food.

'Ha ha! Can't you stop going on about that?' the girl next to me said, and I wondered if she'd lost her mind and was now talking to herself.

I then realised that she was messaging the guy on the other side of the table and I got paranoid. Were they talking about me? Were they slagging me off?

'I think I'll make a move,' I said wearily, thinking about the long journey home on the tube and how I never wore heels anymore because they set the soles of my feet on fire.

'Don't forget your goodie bag,' the PR woman said as I got up to leave.

She handed me an enormous hessian sack with DVDs inside. I wasn't even that excited at this free gift because it was just at the point where DVDs were basically becoming redundant as everyone was streaming everything. I didn't want to seem ungrateful though, so I thanked her and left.

I tell you this story because I often have people asking me if Instagram parties are glamorous and exciting. What I've described wasn't one of those parties, but the feeling I took away was pretty much the same. Ultimately, I felt like there were lots of people out there who were more successful, more technically savvy, more youthful, more famous, more talented and more EVERYTHING than me. It's the same feeling you get if you scroll through Instagram and you're in a bad mood. It just amplifies that mood and you end up getting into more of a funk. The one positive thing I've taken away from getting up close and personal with this world is that beneath the filters and the curated homes are normal people with their own insecurities and their own ups and downs. This is reassuring and a good thing to remember if social media makes you feel like you're lacking in some way.

The alphabet of ageing

A is for Anger, which comes out of nowhere.

B is for Breathing, which is easy to forget to do properly and really helps with the anger.

C is for Comparison, which isn't healthy. It's also for CBD oil which everyone seems to be necking these days.

D is for Depression, which comes and goes, and sometimes just comes and stays.

E is for Elasticated waistbands.

F is for 'FOR FUCK'S SAKE'.

G is for *Golden Girls*, the American TV show. (We're not quite there yet, but we can relate to it more, right?)

H is for Hairy chins and Harry Styles and Hunky (because nobody uses that word anymore).

I is for 'I finally know what I want from life now'.

J is for Junk, which is taking over the loft/shed/house.

K is for Kimchi, which is one of those annoying foods that you don't understand.

L is for Lovely (just to balance out the bollocks and 'for fuck's sake').

M is for Menopause (no longer the thing that happens to your friend's mum).

N is for 'NO' – the power to say 'no' to stuff you don't want. It's also for Netflix, which eats up massive amounts of your time.

O is for Online dungaree ordering, which is an obsession.

P is for 'PUMP UP THE JAM', which was a really good song but now sounds very dated.

Q is for Queens of the Stone Age, which was the last band you went to see live (ten years ago).

R is for Relevant, which is how you want to feel.

S is for Sardines, which are supposed to be very good for your health in your forties.

T is for TV, which is your reason to live.

U is for the U-bend of happiness, which is why you may be unhappy now but will be happier when you're fifty.

V is for Volatile, which is how modern life is.

W is for WOMAN (because you're clearly not a girl).

X is for X-rated thoughts about Cillian Murphy, which are perfectly healthy and normal.

Y is for 'YOU'VE GOT THIS' (and you have).

Z is for Zonked, which is how many of us are made to feel after a day of being judged, trying hard, keeping going, staying youthful (but not too youthful), being made to feel invisible, etc.

Celebrity men ageing versus celebrity women

It's funny, I was looking through some of the coverage of the Johnny Depp court sessions at the Old Bailey and I noticed a few things. First off, there was little reference to Depp's age (fifty-seven). Nor was there much reference to his appearance, which is eccentric to say the least (eyeliner/straw hat/90s bandanna as a face mask). And I was thinking about how the case would have been differently reported if Madonna had been the one turning up for court each day. This is the kind of coverage I'd expect:

Today a smooth, even toned, full-lipped Madonna (aged sixty) walked into court showcasing her incredibly muscular arms, in a cropped top and form-fitting leggings. Madonna (aged sixty) says she owes her UNBELIEVABLE physique to regular workouts and a macrobiotic diet. Some fans may feel she is unrecognisable these days, but Madonna (aged sixty – did we mention her age?) states she is into natural remedies and wouldn't consider more radical measures as she feels they are unethical. Madonna entered the court with her undeniably smooth face and told the court…

And so on. The descriptions of Madonna's appearance would have taken up quite a few column inches and we wouldn't yet be talking about what actually happened in court that day, or the evidence, or the witness testimonies. For older women, just like for younger women but maybe even more pronounced, the main focus is on how they look. The elephant in the room is whether they've actually had any work done. The media won't call this out necessarily but will use lots of snarky comments to imply that work *has* been done. The narrative around older men is quite different. In Depp's case, his appearance isn't mentioned in great detail – certainly the quality of his skin isn't commented on; in fact, his boozed-up, drug-taking antics have been reported as if they're admirable – there is an aura of macho bravado rather than feeling pity or judging. I'm not saying we *should* judge, but it would be a different story if Madonna was up in court, because we'd be reading about how she is an unfit mother, trying to 'cling onto her lost youth' or some other guff about how older women essentially want to be young and any behaviour they exhibit is a manifestation of this. (I know not everyone is on board with how Madonna looks now, but I feel she can do WHATEVER she likes because she is MADONNA and not a regular person like everyone else.)

If we think about Rod Stewart and Paul Weller and Mick Jagger and Ronnie Wood, there isn't much comment made on how their faces have aged or not aged. When Paul Weller launches an album, they don't kick off the interview by saying: 'Paul Weller (sixty-two) has a lived-in face and says he is against cosmeceuticals for ethical reasons and works out about three times a week.' They instead get straight to the album release and what a genius he is and how he has had hit albums every decade for the last five decades. They don't mention the fact that he became a father for the eighth time, aged fifty-nine, which would be the key focus for a female celeb. Equally, people don't describe Ronnie Wood's face and say it looks 'tired and worn out'. However, if Carol Vorderman had aged in a similar way, there would be lots of snarky comments about how 'tired and stressed' she looked.

Okay, this is nothing new. Women are more harshly judged than men when it comes to appearance, but it isn't just appearance.

It's behaviour, too. Men can continue taking drugs, drinking, becoming fathers whenever they like, having wrinkled faces, smoking, having daft haircuts, dating much younger women, bringing out albums, abandoning families and starting new ones, and there is far more leniency from the media. Of course, behind the scenes, they may get up in the morning and rub 'superfood face serum' on their necks and fret that their hair is perhaps a bit silly for a man in his seventies but they can be confident that the media won't unpick their appearance to pieces. There is also quite a bit of romanticism around the older, hedonistic man. He's an archetype. I have lost count of the amount of times I've watched documentaries about Oliver Reed or Peter Cook or Keith Richards, and the drinking and drug taking are seen as admirable, manly and heroic. Let's say Carol Vorderman (I keep coming back to her, I know, but she is often treated in a snarky way by the media) decided to drink whisky all night in a bar and then exited at three in the morning with a younger woman and had a fag hanging out of her mouth and looked dishevelled with maybe some beads tied into her plaited hair (like Richards), would she be held up as an example of heroic, admirable hedonism? Or would we (I mean the culture, us and the media) be thinking that she is 'grasping at her lost youth' or going through a 'mid-life crisis' or 'a mother behaving irresponsibly'. I am not anticipating that Vorderman will suddenly morph into a hedonistic, older rock star, but it feels like this option isn't available to her. She has to look smiley and positive and responsible, and age in an appropriate way that we all feel comfortable with.

I'm not arguing that all older women should be able to snort coke and have funny, beaded hair and leather trousers; but if they choose this path, can we just treat them the same as older men? And can we perhaps stop talking about their appearance quite so much, or if we do talk about it, can we showcase men's appearance in the same way? I would actually be interested in reading about

Paul Weller's skincare regime (I once saw him in an airport in Los Angeles and he was buying anti-ageing cream, and I tried to look over his shoulder to see what he was buying). Now maybe Paul wants advice on how to fight sun damage and the impact of long-term smoking on his eye bags. Or maybe he's not interested because he has more important things to talk about. And there's the rub: he can be older and have more important things to talk about and not have his appearance commented on, or his reproductive life unpicked *because he's a man*.

Why I want to go to Glastonbury but also don't

I feel like Glastonbury has become one of those things that we feel we have to have been to at least once in our lives. If you've never been, people don't see you as a fully rounded individual. It means you can't join in with the stories that people blah on about. You know, the story of how they got lost in a field and ended up taking mushrooms and talking to a strange man for two hours and it turned out to be Joe Strummer from The Clash; or when they crawled into a tent in the middle of the night only to realise that it wasn't their tent and there was actually a performing lion in there that could have eaten them alive. Those kind of stories. Each year I sit on the sofa eating Doritos and watching the TV version, and I say out loud, 'Next year I am going to get tickets. Next year I will register and we will all have to log on to the portal and then we will definitely get tickets, because if there's one thing I need to do before I die it's to go to Glastonbury.' Then this year (2020), Glastonbury was called off due to coronavirus. So instead, there was loads of TV coverage of the best bits of Glastonbury from over the years. The more I watched, the more I realised I would have to attend once.

My issue is this... as I've got older I've learnt that whenever I have big expectations of ANYTHING, it will end up being a disappointment. I used to travel to New York quite a lot for work and I remember the time I booked this flashy hotel in the Meatpacking district. I'd visualised hanging out in the penthouse bar and how there'd be rock stars and models drinking cocktails and I'd be looking cool and collected with my stimulus bag full of advertising for herbal tea packaging concepts (this was what I was researching at the time). Instead, yes, I did stay in a wonderful hotel, but on the Friday night I was too scared to go to the bar on my own, so I walked to the corner shop, got a couple of beers, then waited by the lift with all the glamorous people travelling up to the bar and I went back to my room and watched *Dog the Bounty Hunter* whilst eating a room-service burger with fries. The room had no curtains and I clearly remember my reflection in the glass window, the night time New York skyline in the background – me in my tracksuit pants and my top rolled up, rubbing my tummy, with the TV giving my face an eerie, blue glow. So, the expectation was one thing. Reality was something else.

I could give you millions of other examples of nights out where I've got really dressed up, thinking it would be the BEST NIGHT OF MY ENTIRE LIFE, and then it being okay – not awful but not brilliant either, and usually nowhere near what I'd hoped it would be.

So, my fear with Glastonbury is that my expectations are very high. I envisage myself wearing the perfect outfit, which would be something that a fat Kate Moss would wear – definitely with sequins and feathers. I'd be in the VIP area sipping something glamorous and smoking a doobie but definitely nothing too full-on and not gurning. I'd be in conversation with Dave Grohl and telling him about my experience in New York, and he'd be laughing really loudly (and possibly considering whether to ask me then and there to marry him or whether to save it up for when Coldplay came on). I'd have possibly left my children at home because I've never fantasised about going to a festival with children.

(I don't care how many parents tell me it's okay and there is kids' face painting and you can drag them around in one of those trendy pull-along wagons. I DO NOT WANT TO GO TO A MUSIC FESTIVAL WITH SMALL CHILDREN.) Anyway, back to my fantasy, and I'm just a tiny bit stoned and drinking this cocktail and entertaining various attractive rock stars and being flirtatious (but only mildly so) and at some point I'm able to hear the bands on stage perfectly because I'm near the stage (I'm actually in that bit that you see when they film the band – the bit up by the side where the real show-offs go, the friends of the band) and there will be a few cutaway shots of me now and then as I nod my head and laugh and Dave asks me whether I want more doobie or not.

You can see my expectations are VERY HIGH. And so, what will the real Glastonbury experience be like? Will it manage to deliver? I am thinking it may not. And you are thinking HOW COULD IT? And so I am thinking that maybe I should just pretend that I've been, and when people swap their Glastonbury stories, I should just make something up about how I got lost in a disco tent and woke up next to Carl Barât, and be done with it. Nobody needs to know the truth, do they?

Ten things I thought I would be able to do when I got older

It's funny. My eldest daughter was talking to me yesterday and she said, 'Mum, I can't wait until I'm eighteen and can do whatever I want and don't have to go to bed when you say and can watch as much YOUTUBE as I want. It's going to be brilliant.'

I looked at her flushed and excited face and felt sad. It's only with the benefit of hindsight that I can see that childhood is in fact THE BEST TIME EVER. A time when anything is possible. When someone gives you a set routine and you don't have to worry about whether you're making the right life choices. She's six at the moment, and I can remember feeling the same way when I was a child. I couldn't wait to get shot of my parents and run off into the world. I believed that adulthood would deliver me into this idyllic place (mainly idyllic because nobody would be telling me what to do). I had a whole heap of expectations of the things I'd be able to do once I was a proper adult. In my twenties I still didn't feel like a proper adult, and when I reflect on it now, I spent much of the time apologising for my existence and feeling like I was worthless. Then in my thirties I got more confident but still lived my life like a weird adult–child hybrid, working and being serious by day, and drinking and pretending I was in my twenties by night. Now I'm in my late forties and I still don't feel like an adult. These are some of the things I thought I'd be able to do but still can't:

1. Cook a meal without burning/boiling to death/spoiling one element.
2. Be able to drive on a motorway.
3. Provide healthy snacks for my children (good things like chopped-up fruit and vegetables, not crisps, sweets or an old mashed-up banana with a wet wipe stuck to it) that are in a Tupperware box.
4. Be able to look at a man that I fancy and not blush.
5. Understand politics.
6. Always have tissues/wipes/lip balm/hair bands/sun screen/change of clothes/nappies/hair brush/water/purse/mobile charger in my bag and not ALWAYS HAVE ONE THING – USUALLY THE MOST VITAL THING – MISSING.
7. Exit a toilet without having my skirt tucked into my tights.
8. Be able to do the 'black, winged eyeliner' thing. I have read upwards of fifteen articles on how to do this but still can't.

9. Have the willpower to not snack in front of the TV and watch shit, and not read celebrity interviews in magazines and feel insecure and crap because I'm not a size 8 and don't live in an eight-bedroom house with a giant kitchen and walk-in wardrobes.

10. Get somewhere in a hurry without falling over.

CHAPTER THIRTEEN

How It Took Me Forty-Seven Years to Learn
That Buying Stuff Isn't a Route to Happiness

I grew up with a feminist step-mum, mum, and a dad who was a Marxist. They called me Anniki because it sounded like ANARCHY and my dad wanted to sock it to 'the man'. He was horrified by 1980s consumerism, and laughed like a drain whenever Maggie Thatcher was ridiculed on the *Spitting Image* TV show. Growing up, we had many arguments in the supermarket because I'd want to buy Coco Pops and he would dissect the packaging, and rant about how it represented 'obscene capitalist ideology', and then he'd buy this super-un-tasty, worthy muesli which you had to chew for half an hour before you could swallow it. I'd emerge from Sainsbury's in tears and promise myself that the moment I left home I'd eat Coco Pops all the time and buy proper washing detergent that cleaned the stains out of your clothes rather than the peculiar hemp-seed/lavender guff we got in the wholefood shop.

My parents were trying to make a difference. They wanted the world to be a better place. Dad went to South Africa and campaigned against apartheid (he was a treasurer for the UDF – an affiliate organisation of the ANC). Mum volunteered in Nicaragua. They did not buy Coco Pops. They didn't let me watch crap on TV (well, sometimes I watched *A-Team* and *Knight Rider*, but that was a special treat). My dad's favourite refrain when he entered the room and the TV was on was 'What's this capitalist crap then?' They didn't buy more than they needed. Mum liked to buy second-hand everything, and her favourite activity was to schlep around antique shops looking for old cupboards she could paint and transform (this was before all the trendy 'upcycling' stuff). I wanted clothes from Next, and Timberland boots, like my friends'. I remember people laughing at me in my dorky pinafore dress and sandals.

My parents wanted me to inherit some of these recycling, non-conformist, values. Did I take these on board? In a word, No.

The moment I had proper money (when I got my job in market research, the job that I stayed in most of my life), I developed an obsession with buying clothes. I believed that a new outfit would deliver me a spanking new future. I wasn't sure how this would happen, but standing in Top Shop once a week, my brain would light up and I'd project myself, wearing the new shirt/dress/jumper, and I'd be a happier, more lovable version of myself. Everything would be brilliant.

Why did I believe this? Because it was what advertising taught me (and, yes, I was one of the people selling this idea). I also believed that using an anti-cellulite cream made by monks in a tiny monastery in the Dordogne would make my legs look like Cindy Crawford's. I was addicted to women's magazines and bought a copy of French *Vogue* when I was fourteen. It cost £4 and was as thick as a brick. I looked at all those beautiful women and realised with sadness I'd never be one of them. I desperately wanted to be a model. Models had perfect lives where they were transported on clouds whilst being fed grapes by handsome pop stars.

I couldn't be a model but I sort of believed that wearing nice clothes, new clothes, ever-changing clothes, would elevate my life in a similar way. It sounds sad, right? At the top of my game, when I was earning a lot of money (remember it took me twelve years to ascend the greasy pole), I'd walk into Selfridges and go up to the clothing floor (it was always high-street fashion that I binged on – I never bought designer clothing, which was just as well as

I would have been bankrupt), and I'd walk around with my arms laden down with clothes and bump into other women – tired, stressed, fucked-off women – doing exactly the same (has it ever struck you that people who are buying mountains of stuff don't look very happy?). The stupid thing was, I didn't have any occasion to wear these clothes. I spent the majority of my time sitting in badly-lit viewing facilities, furnished with beige furniture and clichéd images of birds flying and mountain views, moderating hours of group discussions whilst impatient clients sat behind a mirror and chiefly talked about how tired they were, and how their flights had been delayed for hours, and how they hated the food that had been provided because it wasn't macrobiotic. I travelled to lots of different countries for work, and in those countries I usually bought more clothes. I often couldn't shut my suitcase because it was so stuffed with booty. I wore my new clothes whilst moderating groups on dog biscuits and loo rolls, and they gave me the illusion that my life was successful and glamorous.

And yes, of course, a nice item of clothing can make you feel better about life. I'm not saying that we have to walk about in our pants and bras, beating ourselves with birch branches all day, but it's more about trying to be more mindful and thinking: *What is going on with me right now. Do I need to buy these dungarees? Why am I online shopping in this moment? Is it because I've had a shit day and feel like I've been rubbish at parenting and made a faux pas in an email?* (i.e. acknowledging that spending is usually linked to something that's going on in a broader context or is something we use to perk us up when we're emotionally low).

We know that rich people with lots of stuff aren't happy. We see it in the faces of the Kardashian family. There is a *lack* – a sense that they have EVERYTHING on a material level but are still miserable and as insecure as fuck. The fact that they fly on private planes and have massive walk-in wardrobes that look like boutique fashion stores doesn't stop them arguing about who is the prettiest or who has the best style or who has the most followers. It took me forty-seven years to understand that buying stuff isn't a route to happiness. As I got older, the desire for clothes transformed into a desire to have a kitchen extension (the same kitchen extension that everybody has, with the same island in the middle and the tap that pours boiling water out of it so you don't have to boil the kettle). I then realised that I do most of my thinking when the kettle is boiling and what have we come to if we can't wait a minute for a cup of tea? I also wanted that box on the top of my house – the one that said to the world that I was successful and had arrived. If I had these things, I'd be happy.

Then the coronavirus crisis kicked off, Dad died, and life changed. I worried less about the luxury of having more space and worried about whether the people I loved would die. I looked at my wardrobe and realised it belonged to a gluttonous, numpty – a numpty who thought nice clothes would make her life perfect... It made me think differently about the way I consume and, more importantly, how consuming stuff won't stop me ageing, or help me fight death. Yes, buying a jumpsuit can give me a momentary thrill (and I'm not completely weaned off shopping), but I don't feel the same about buying things now. I know that shopping won't make my life better (unless it's a new washing machine). I've sat in a new jumpsuit and cried because I miss my dad. I have also worn lovely face cream and worried about the future and what our lives will look like once coronavirus calms down (if it calms down – it will calm down, right?).

'I went to TK Maxx yesterday, and I just thought, "What is all this stuff?"' a friend said to me recently, gesturing around hopelessly. 'I was like, "WHO NEEDS IT? DOES ANYONE NEED IT NOW?"' She shook her head.

'I feel like we need to spend in order to get things back to normal. I mean that was our life, right? Earning money and spending it?' I said.

'Yes,' she said. 'A few months ago, and I would have come out with a whole load of things, but it just feels wrong now. It doesn't feel the same. The fun has gone.'

Coronavirus has not only shaken things up on a macro level, making us think about our values and what's most important, it has also schooled us on how little we miss going to the shops perhaps? For me there is this additional layer of age and the realisation that buying clothes won't fill the void. It won't make me feel better. If anything, it just makes me feel guilty (and let's consider the ethical dimension of rampant consumerism – the fact that we're destroying the planet in the process). I have enough stuff. I would like a bigger house but I know that having a bigger house won't make me happy long term (there is actually something called the 'hedonic treadmill', which means we quickly assimilate whatever we have and then want more). I want to be more in control of my finances as I've never really managed to work to a budget and have always told myself that I was rubbish at money (this has meant that I live in fear whenever I check my bank balance as I don't feel empowered enough to manage a budget).

So, how do we cut back when we've been programmed to believe that buying things makes our lives better? How do we stop? How do we realise that spending all the time doesn't make us happy? As I move towards my fifth decade, I am thinking differently about the way I consume stuff and am cutting back.

I spoke to Clare Seal, creator of the 'My Frugal Year' Instagram account and author of *Real Life Money: An Honest Guide to Taking Control of Your Finances.* Clare found herself in £27k of debt overall and decided to act:

> It was a case of when we're earning more, we will pay it back; or, when I get my bonus, we will pay it back. It was always a problem for later. Last March we got to the middle of the month and I was in an unplanned overdraft and the bank advisor asked me when

I'd come back to my limit, and I said, 'Well, that'll be pay day,' and I heard myself say the words 'There is just no money left.'

The thing is, we often have a lot of residual fear around money as women and tend to take a passive approach – not checking our balance, feeling guilty when we buy stuff, and ultimately telling ourselves that money isn't something we're 'good at'. Women are educated to believe that finances and money aren't in their control. They are also on the backfoot finance-wise because they earn less than their male counterparts. Clare says:

> It's really strange, a lot of it stems from the triple bind that women find themselves in. The historical culture around money. Women are paid less and the gender pay gap isn't closing fast enough. That's before we talk about having children or caring for older relatives, as women make up the majority of carers. We are losing out. From a young age, we're told that the most important thing is how we look and that there is something wrong with us in our natural state – we're too fat or too thin and our hair isn't the right colour. We are then flogged stuff to fix that.

We are taught that in order to be attractive, successful women, to fit in with society and be liked and respected, we need to have a lot of tools, potions, clothes, shoes, accessories and consumer goods.

The link between buying stuff and feeling better about ourselves

The problem is that buying stuff doesn't make us feel good. There is a momentary lift as we grab the thing and have it in our hands and march to the till, but that lift soon fades as we walk out of the shop and feel guilt or worry that we shouldn't have bought that thing/

didn't need it/have acted too impetuously. There are, of course, times when buying stuff is fulfilling – it's just that women are often trapped in a cycle of buying things as one of the ONLY ways of feeling better or escaping uncomfortable feelings (i.e. buying loads of clothes because they are miserable in a relationship/job/life in general). When we get older, this buying stuff thing can continue, but the stuff changes, so instead of clothes it could be a kitchen extension or fancy holidays or posh dinners out. Ultimately, it will be the kind of blanket we wear in the retirement home and whether it's the right brand of slipper we shuffle about in. Once we get on the consumerist treadmill, it's very hard to get off.

How to tackle your relationship with money and face the music

Not all of us will get into debt, but many of us are spending more than we want to or simply don't feel in control of our money. I often talk to friends and they'll say things like 'God, I just found myself buying these trainers and I don't even need them but I got them anyway'. There is a searching for approval in their tone, a sense of 'Yes I know I shouldn't do this, but actually it's okay, right, because we all do this and buy stuff we don't need, right?'

We are used to being painted as people who can't control spending, and there are plentiful examples in films and TV that show women as hapless spenders, surrounded by shopping bags, unable to stop, but it's actually okay because it's fun! (*Sex and the City* was one of those shows that seemed to show an awful lot of shopping, depicting it as a way to bond with friends – maybe the main way of bonding, along with drinking cocktails.)

If you want to tackle your finances and understand your spending, then it's about starting that journey and acknowledging that things aren't as you want them to be. Clare says that progress is rarely linear and that sometimes tackling our relationship with money happens in fits and starts. It can feel like you're failing, but for some people it's a journey of awareness and taking it at your own pace:

> For some people, getting everything out at once helps. I checked my balances bit by bit and my credit score bit by bit, and called my bank and lenders because I knew that if I tried to do it all in one day, I would frighten myself and put my head back in the sand. We all know ourselves, and if we think about events in our lives, we know how we respond. So the big thing is, if you are at the point, then don't try and use a prescription that someone else has written. And also, don't feel bad if something goes wrong one month – you're more likely to spiral out of control again.

Be practical and start with a budget

One of the best things to do is to shop with a budget. So instead of worrying about how much you've spent, have a clear budget in mind for something and know that you're shopping within it. It sounds simple, but many women still shy away from this approach and don't face up to their spending. Clare says:

> The best way to do it is to live with a budget so you know what's going in and coming out and what you want to do with it. That's all a budget is, and usually on a Sunday I take half an hour and look at all those things.

Ultimately, as we get older, it's important that we feel in touch with why we're spending, and don't let it control us. This is especially true when so many products and brands target older women and offer up 'solutions' to ageing. I always notice that I buy 'anti-ageing' face cream if I'm tired and worn out and have had a bad day. I am especially vulnerable to buying clothes if I feel bored and dissatisfied with my life or like stuff is passing me by (Instagram is especially dangerous for this as I tend to scroll and then hit directly on links and buy stuff because I feel like my life isn't as great as the person I'm following). The more power we have over our spending means the more power we have over our money, which translates into more power over our lives. It has taken me a long time to realise this. I am still learning it now. I am not immune to feeling jealous of a kitchen extension or a nice pair of trainers, but I am getting better and planning and thinking about WHY I long for these things.

And the adage that you can never have enough clothes is not true. You can definitely have enough clothes.

I have anyway.

Tips on how to react when women get competitive and downright rude

It's funny, but competition between women isn't talked about much. Having spent years in the company of women, and working with them, and being friends with them, and standing at the school gates with them, I've found that we're all complex bitches. Why do we feel the need to compete? We feel the need because we've been raised to see our fellow women as barriers to our happiness. We think that we will feel better if we put another woman down. Or we just feel resentful because they have a bigger house and it gets on our nerves. I would like to say that when women get competitive, I back off and do some meditation instead, but sometimes, to be completely honest, I wish I could be more direct. This is especially true as I've got older and more aware of how subservient I can become and how I need to step up my game. Yes, in an ideal world there would be nothing but camaraderie and love between women, but let's cut the shit and be authentic and flag up that sometimes women are rude and horrible to one another and that isn't going to stop. So, these are my dream responses to typical scenarios that you might come across when a woman is being rude and competitive (either/or).

SCENARIO ONE
Someone is boasting about their holiday plans, despite knowing that you're skint and will have to spend the summer sitting in the local park eating stale Dairylea dunker crackers out of your

rucksack, picking fag butts out of the sandpit and helping a toddler get on the slide and off the slide and on the slide and off again until you want to die.

Rude woman: Well we're flying straight to Tuscany and then we have our own villa but we've hired a Land Rover and will be exploring the locality and we're taking our nanny with us so we can get some chill time because we're exhausted after our last holiday, which was the one in New York without the kids that I told you about last time I was talking down to you in the park.

You have two choices here. You can go for the direct approach or try something a little more sophisticated. I've presented both.

Option one: Bye! I have a meeting with Anna Wintour about my new over-forties fashion line for size 16+ women – we're doing a Zoom that starts in ten minutes! She is sponsoring the line and I'll be on the cover of *Vogue* next month.

Option two: Oh dear, I've heard there's a snail plague in Tuscany and people are getting boils on their faces because of the snails that have been let loose. It's really fucking up peoples' holidays but hey… maybe you'll luck out and the plague will have finished by the time you get there.

The latter option is tricky. In fact, they are both tricky because you're lying and will be found out, but as long as you never see this person again, it's fine.

SCENARIO TWO

You're talking to someone about your kid and how hard it is to entertain them sometimes and how you're feeling overwhelmed and don't know how everyone else does it. You're really hoping for some honesty but you don't get it – in fact, quite the opposite.

Rude woman: Well, we don't allow any screen time. I like the kids to be free-range, so we have this beautiful worm farm and they play with it for hours. We do yoga as the sun comes up and then I like to check on the sourdough to see how it's developing. In the afternoon we collect feathers and grind them up to make our very own 'feather insect paste', which we then daub on the worm farm to attract moths and other creatures, which we do pencil drawings of until it's bedtime. We listen to whale sounds and they sleep in my arms.

Option one: Well, it's funny you said 'worms', because we covered the whole worm farm thing last year but have moved on and have turned our food compost bin into an eco-farm and the children have named all the maggots and we've made clothes for them out of tiny pieces of egg shell. I guess worm farms were more popular last year. Then in the afternoon we go paddle boarding on the canal and then camp up in the field. I mean who needs sleep anyway?

Option two: It's funny but I think screens are excellent. In the future we will have these helmets beaming content directly into our eyes, so I want my kids to be ready and be great at coding. But I guess if you want to live in the past with the worms, then that's fine, right?

Neither of these responses are very nice, but you don't have to be nice if someone is making you feel bad. Being nice is not going to make you feel better in the short term.

SCENARIO THREE

You're at an influencer event and you tell someone your book idea and they look down their nose at you, and then sigh – a sigh that makes you feel like your new idea is a bucket of panda shit.

Rude woman: Well, I've written a book with @Happymum-mylove and we got an advance of £100k each and we've just had it optioned by Channel 4, and Sharon Horgan is directing it – you like her, right, but we're best buds. She's HILARIOUS but she apparently thinks you're stalking her on Instagram. Anyway, I've heard that books about ageing are a bit commonplace, so you might need to rethink your strategy. You don't know @Happymummylove, right? We did an amazing glamping trip last year, but they only invited influencers with over 100,000 followers. Must be off. Fearne Cotton has just walked in and I'm on her podcast soon.

Option one: Fuck off.

Option two: @Happymummylove told me you had herpes and that she hates you, and also Sharon Horgan texted me to say you're a hateful person and she doesn't want to direct your show because it's nonsense and you only got a deal because you're an influencer. And I've already done Fearne's podcast and we do play dates every weekend, so I'll have to be off now as she wants to leave so we can hang out together and make vegan cupcakes and chat with Russell Brand about positive visualisation.

Again, this response relies on several factors – you can never see this person again, or @Happymummlove again, or Sharon Horgan, or Fearne Cotton, because all of them will know you are a liar. You may also jeopardise any book deal you could have got, because everyone will know you're a horrible liar and rumours will circulate and you may have to move home and come off all social media. So perhaps just do option one instead.

CHAPTER FOURTEEN

Advice on the Next Twenty-Five+ Years of Your Life

*How to Learn to Embrace Getting Older and
the 'Crunchy Times' Ahead*

A few months back, I went for a massage and the masseuse said to me, 'Wow you have a crunchy neck.' And this is what growing older is about. It's about THE CRUNCHY NECK but also about the CRUNCHY TIMES – a whole confluence of factors:

Physical: feeling tired and depleted; unable to cope with hangovers; experiencing the menopause.
Emotional: feeling less relevant and less in the game; more prone to anxiety and worry; feeling like the best years are behind us.

It's CRUNCHY, and no amount of light massage will dispatch those feelings. In my survey there is an underlying desire to feel different, to know that confidence *should* be the end game, but this is just a sugar coating, a thing we say, and underneath the wobbles persist:

I remember finding it funny at the time, seeing myself as a 'gonna-be', with my whole life in front of me. Seeing it again is like a dagger to the heart ;) What happened? How did I get here? But also wanting to age gracefully and embrace where I am.

Why the fuck did it take this long for me to get here and worry about life choices/opportunities at work/dilemmas? Having to consider what's most important to me (kids, work, relationship, friends, etc.). Suddenly being one of the oldest at work! Feeling like a bit of a has-been.

I feel getting older isn't really an option for women. We are expected to find ways to keep ourselves looking young. I certainly don't feel that an older women is celebrated in any way.

But what would change look like? Well it means more than a couple of fluffy interviews with celebrity women sprouting on about CONFIDENCE and not sharing any of the challenges. It's also not just paying lip service to older women by throwing them the odd bone now and then (i.e. let's have more TV and content that focuses on older women, rather than the odd exception here and there). Oh, and it also means more than putting one grey-haired woman in an advertising campaign and feeling like you've ticked the box for another few months. Of course there are many things that need to change that are not age-related – our relationship with the planet, with our fellow humans and with consumerism are all things that need to be challenged, but what about how we age and ensuring that we aren't spending the final few decades of our lives worrying and ruminating because we're not feeling like a jubilant model in a Tena-lady advert?

Much of my life I've projected forwards, so thinking…

When I'm in my twenties I'll be happy because I'll have a proper job and be able to buy stuff and will finally be able to drive a car.

No, hang on, when I'm thirty I'll be happy because I'll have more money and my own house and will finally be able to drive a car.

Wait, I'll be happy in my forties because I'll have children and a kitchen extension and nice holidays and will finally be able to drive a car.

I can drive a car now but I haven't driven since I passed my test because I'm too scared. I'm scared that I'll crash, scared that if I go on the motorway I'll never be able to get off, scared that I will drive over a cliff edge and never be seen again. And this creates an interesting analogy with ageing. As a forty-seven-year-old woman, I've officially 'passed my test' (i.e. I know the things that make me happy and all the stuff that makes me feel shit) but I am still too scared to GET IN THE CAR AND DRIVE.

What do I mean? I mean being in charge of our own destiny and not letting culture and society shape how we feel about ageing. We need to slow down if necessary, because there is no need to stay in the fast lane unless you want to (personally, I find it's fucking exhausting). We need to not focus on the other cars flying past and not worry about how much shinier they are and how our own vehicle is a bit of a mess and has a decaying McDonald's Happy Meal mushed up in the back seat and two children mewling that they need the toilet. We need to know when it's okay to sit behind a lumbering lorry and when we need to indicate, pull out and hit the accelerator. Okay, I'm going to stop with the driving analogy, but we need to have agency. And whilst there are still some basic rules (like don't crash into other cars or drive in the opposite direction – sorry I can't stop this), the route that you choose is yours. This is where the driving thing ends, because actually you can mount the pavement if you like, go up into the hills, slow down or go fast. But whatever you do, don't continue to be someone you think you *should* be instead of the person you are.

I always remember that famous scene in *Thelma & Louise* where they fly off into oblivion at the end of the movie (sorry if I've spoilt it for you, but you must have seen it already). I think that's how I want ageing to feel – that's how I want the next chapter of my life to be. I want to be jumping into the unknown (not death though, ideally) and feel that same sense of being entirely carefree and not projecting forward anymore; because the truth is, life cannot be put off any longer once you get to your forties. My dad died just a couple of months shy of his retirement. I had certain idealised visions of what his life would be like once he gave up work – how he would read books, write books, be available to play with and look after my daughters who adored him, how we'd go on holidays together, how he'd explain all the big life events we'd been through together (especially the death of my step-mum and sister, which we'd never discussed), and then he'd teach me about philosophy because I was always too impatient and self-absorbed to listen when I was a teenager. And none of these things happened. And whilst that rips my heart up and makes me feel panicked, it also reminds me that life cannot be put off any longer. Although I don't want to jump about the beach like a fool, I do want to feel that my life makes more sense to me, that there is a balance between good and shit and that I'm not living out the life of someone on fast-forward autopilot.

The one truism about ageing (no matter how you choose to do it) is that you are closer to death. If you can remember that fact, it can actually be quite liberating, because other stuff falls to the side. If you really think that there are maybe 25–30 years left, then that's not very long is it? That doesn't mean you have to accomplish more things and be productive but it does mean you have to find out who you are and do more of the things that make you happy. So, on a very simple level, it's about thinking about what you want from life. If we cannot finally say what we want, then when will that time come? I'm imagining this kind of scenario:

LOCATION: A RETIREMENT HOME IN RURAL SOMERSET

Anniki: Do you think this amount of blusher is inappropriate for someone my age?

Carer: You're eighty-five, Anniki. I think you can do whatever the hell you want.

Anniki: [Pointing at shoes.] No, but seriously, I read that I'm supposed to never wear socks with trainers. It says it in the *Style* supplement. I have to wear those invisible socks apparently.

Carer: But who's going to know?

Anniki: Society? Culture? God?

Carer: [Growing frustrated.] We're going to start the chair aerobics session in a bit and I really don't think it matters.

Anniki: [Sadly.] I don't think chair aerobics is something a woman my age should be doing. My pelvic floor is destroyed post-kids. I've got four podcasts I need to listen to and then some Ted Talks that I'm supposed to catch up on.

Carer: They're not called 'podcasts', Anniki. They're called 'Zimbowacks' and you'll need the avatar-enhanced AI machine but it's busted. Anyway, you were telling me yesterday that you'd written a book in 2020 and the main theme was THERE ARE NO RULES TO AGEING AND YOU CAN DO EXACTLY WHAT YOU LIKE.

Anniki: Oh yeah. I forgot. It was the same year we had that coronavirus pandemic. Have you seen my glasses anywhere by the way?

Carer: They're in your lap. What's up? You look sad.

Anniki: I'd forgotten about the book. I'd forgotten that society is telling me what I can and can't do but actually I can do whatever I want. I'm going to get my tie-dye kaftan out and wear it to dinner tonight. I kept worrying it was too ageing, but you're right!

Carer: Great. We have a Radiohead tribute band tomorrow lunchtime.

Anniki: God, I love them. I wonder if it'll be as good as the Massive Attack one that was on last month.

Anniki wanders off to find her kaftan but by the time she reaches her wardrobe she's forgotten that she can do whatever she wants and so has to go and speak to the carer, who hands her a copy of her book which is dog-eared and falling apart.

So, you're in your forties now. Or you're coming up to fifty? Or maybe even sixty? WHOSE PERMISSION ARE YOU WAITING FOR? If you want me to give you permission, then here you go:

Dear Reader,

You officially have permission to do what you want, look how you want, say what you want (as long as you're not offending or hurting anyone), work how you want, mother how you want (again as long as you've got the bases covered), and there is little point in paying attention to what society deems is fitting for an older woman or what employers think is a good fit or what fashion writers think. You can wear socks with trainers. You can change careers. You can have Botox or think it's repulsive. You can have pink hair. Wear a kaftan. Listen to Stormzy. You can be confident one day and feel like a sack of shit the next. It's not enough to just be alive (going back to the first chapter of this book and how we are made to feel lucky just to be older – yes okay, but mere survival is not enough).

Love Anniki x

And here is an ode to all of you, you know who you are

And you, with the grey hair struggling to get a screaming toddler into a car seat, I salute you.

You, with the aching back, squinting into a laptop, trying to design your new website, I salute you.

You, waking in the night covered in sweat and fear and dread, I salute you.

You, losing your dad, or your mum, or your sister, or best friend, I salute you.

You, writing 'fuck off,' in the margin of your exercise book in a work meeting because nobody is listening, I salute you.

You, secretly wishing you could snog someone inappropriate, I salute you.

You, trying to find your glasses, I salute you.

You, crying because you haven't had sex in years, I salute you.

You, watching the 'Live Aid' documentary and wondering where the last twenty years have gone and then realising it is, in fact, thirty-five years, I salute you.

You, thinking the best is behind you, but it isn't. It doesn't have to be.

I *am* you.

And to summarise, some final advice

Yes, I know if you're like me, then you need money and work, but can you find a job that doesn't make you feel second-best? And, yes, if you feel shit about your face, then have Botox, but don't feel guilty. If you don't want it, then don't, but also don't judge women who find it makes them feel better. There are clearly many different routes to ageing. One of them is clearly signposted 'JUDGEMENT, RIGIDITY, ROUTINE' and another is signposted 'NON-JUDGEMENT, FLEXIBILITY, CHANGE'.

The latter is far less ageing in the conventional sense. Don't be the grumpy, bitter person in the corner who is pissed off with her life and her choices. Don't feel like you have to be zippety doo daaah all day either, but remember to keep moving, be open, keep learning and accept change – embrace these things and they will all stand you in good stead.

The How to Be A Boss at Ageing Manifesto

- Don't feel that you're less than brilliant because you're older than everyone else in the room.
- Don't be bossed around by fashion writers who tell you tosh like 'YOU MUST NOT WEAR TRAINERS WITH SOCKS ONCE YOU GET PAST FORTY-FIVE' (this was in an article recently).
- Don't be ashamed of Botox. Don't be bullied into Botox either (by society/friends/whatever).
- If you're not enjoying the party, then leave.
- As Janet Street Porter famously wrote (in her book of the same name), 'Life is too fucking short'. This motto can be applied to most decision making.
- Don't develop a side hustle because you feel you have to do. Do some knitting instead (but don't feel like the knitting has to be a brand that is launched with an event and supports your entire family long term and you're a flop if it doesn't).
- There's no law that dictates what older women should or shouldn't do. Nobody is going to tell you off for dancing to Wu-Tang Clan or smoking a fag.
- (The above is quite liberating.)
- Don't be ashamed if you're the oldest mum on the school run.
- Don't fret about chin hairs. Kate Moss has them too.

- Spend at least an hour a day doing nothing. Don't feel guilty about this.
- Keep trying new things, even if it's just a different topping at Pizza Express.
- Read something that challenges you – politically, spiritually, culturally.
- Find an older woman that inspires you. Copy what she does.
- Look after your body.
- Give up alcohol if the negatives far outweigh any positives.
- Read up on the menopause.
- Have sex if you feel like it. If you don't, then at least do something fun with your partner that is not supermarket shopping.
- Remember to slow down – there's no gold certificate for being the busiest, most stressed woman in the world.
- The best years are yet to come (maybe that's not strictly true, but don't continue to put up with the stuff that drives you mad). Embrace the road ahead. Don't put life off for another minute. Don't let others make you feel bad either. Wear trainers and socks if you want.
- Don't hold back and wait for the right time. I give you permission to get on with it. Not that you need my permission of course.

A LETTER FROM ANNIKI

Dear Reader,

First off, I want to say a MASSIVE thanks for choosing to read *How to Be a Boss at Ageing.* If you enjoyed it, and want to keep up-to-date with all my latest releases, just sign up at the link below. Your email address will never be shared and you can unsubscribe at any time. I know how annoying too many emails can be, believe me!

www.thread-books.com/anniki-sommerville

Why did I write *How to Be a Boss at Ageing*?

Well, first and foremost, I wrote this book for myself. Aged forty-seven, I looked around and realised I was classed as 'middle-aged' and wasn't sure what the future looked like. Was I supposed to just embrace it and prance about on the beach like a lady in an incontinence pad advert? What if I was feeling ambivalent and anxious instead? What would growing older look like in a society that fetishises youth? Was it okay to get tweakments or did it mean you were no longer a feminist? What kind of job could I hope to get and still feel like my skills were relevant? What about my relationship? Was it normal for it to become a mixture of box sets and the odd M&S 'Dine in for Two'? Then I lost my dad at the beginning of lockdown. He died suddenly and it made me question the big picture: if life could finish to quickly, then what would the next chapter of my own life look like? Could I start to differentiate between the stuff that mattered and the stuff that didn't? I started a podcast, and each week interviewed a different expert, covering off themes such as infertility, friendship, motherhood, sex, work, peri-menopause and menopause, anxiety and money.

I started getting messages on my Instagram from women telling me that they were also experiencing problems in their forties – they were feeling invisible, suffering from anxiety, going through the peri-menopause and menopause and were desperate to get their hands on information. So, I did a survey of over 300 women and discovered that many of these feelings were universal. I organised the various topics by chapter and wrote down all my findings, including quotes from the survey, my own personal perspective, and tips and advice from experts in the various fields (as well as people who had experienced something similar). I wanted the book to be informative with tangible tips and advice but also some light relief. I've included lots of fun lists, with a view to dipping in and out of the book whenever you're in need of a mental boost.

I get asked about ageing a lot. It has turned into my specialist subject. The truth is, I'm not an expert but have spoken to lots of people who are. I have realised that a lot of it is about our mindset and preparing ourselves properly. I've spoken to many women who are struggling and looking for some quick and easy ways to improve their lives and see the light at the end of the tunnel. The truth is, the peri-menopause and menopause are no walk in the park; the sense that we are losing our visual currency is also a biggie when we've been brought up to believe that the way we look is a key measure of how successful we are as women. But there *is* light at the end of the tunnel! And there is fun to be had. It's not all bad news. Honestly!

Okay, physically we are undergoing radical changes, and then we have these fundamental mental shifts to contend with, like anxiety. This is without taking into account all the outside pressures that we've felt in the last eighteen months (a pandemic, lockdown, political upheaval, climate change) The thing is, there are plenty of positives to ageing, too: a sense of caring less about what others think, being more aware of our own mortality, which may sound depressing but is important because it helps us prioritise and re-focus on what's important, and being more aware of what we want; there's also a sense of freedom – of being able to finally shape the next chapter of our lives.

I hope you loved the book and I'd love for you to listen to the podcast and join the Facebook support group. We share our experiences and also silly giphys that make us feel better. Ultimately, 'How to Be a Boss at Ageing' is not just a book – it's a movement, and a community with courses and events – all with a view to helping women navigate their forties and fifties and not feel so knackered and hopeless.

I love hearing from my readers – you can get in touch on Instagram, through my Facebook page, Goodreads, or my website.

Thanks, and remember… keep on truckin', don't let the ageing police get you down.

Ask yourself… What do you want your life to look like and what steps are you going to take today to get yourself there?

Anniki x

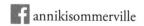 annikisommerville

www.annikisommervilleisworking.com

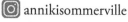 annikisommerville

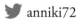 anniki72

Everything That Has Helped Me Navigate My Forties and Beyond... AKA 'Resources'

Books

For no-nonsense beauty advice: *Pretty Honest* by Sali Hughes.

For simple and useful sex advice: *More Orgasms Please: Why Female Pleasure Matters* by The Hotbed Collective; *Mind the Gap* by Dr Karen Gurney.

For when you want to learn more about the history of beauty and how the patriarchy has shaped that history: *The Beauty Myth: How Images of Beauty Are Used Against Women* by Naomi Wolf.

For when you want to learn more about your menstrual cycle: *Wild Power – Discover the Magic of Your Menstrual Cycle and Awaken the Feminine Path to Power* by Alexandra Pope and Sjanie Hugo Wurlitzer; *Period* by Maisie Hill.

For when you're dealing with difficult emotions: *Emotional Agility* by Susan David; *First We Make the Beast Beautiful* by Sarah Wilson; *The Worry Trick: How Your Brain Tricks You into Expecting the Worst and What You Can Do about It* by David A. Carbonell.

For when you feel fed up and need a kick up the bum: *Life's Too Fucking Short* by Janet Street Porter.

For when you're truly knackered and overwhelmed: *A Mindfulness Guide for the Frazzled* by Ruby Wax.

For changing bad habits: *Better Than Before: What I Learned about Making and Breaking Habits* by Gretchen Rubin.

For when you're considering sobriety: *Love Yourself Sober: A Self-Care Guide to Alcohol-Free Living for Busy Mothers* by Mandy Manners and Kate Bailey; *The Unexpected Joy of Being Sober* by Catherine Gray.

For when you can't leave your phone alone: *How to Break Up with Your Phone* by Catherine Price.

For when you're in need of a clever and funny viewpoint on modern life: *Wow No Thank You* by Samantha Irby.

If you want to re-design your work life: *The Freelance Mum* by Annie Ridout; *Flex: The Modern Woman's Handbook* by Annie Auerbach.

If you want to learn more about white privilege: *Why I No Longer Talk to White People about Race* by Reni Eddo-Lodge.

If you want to learn more about racism: *So You Want to Talk about Race* by Ijeoma Oluo.

For menopause (and more) inspiration: *The Shift: How I (lost and) Found Myself after 40 – and You Can Too* by Sam Baker; *The New Hot: Taking on the Menopause with Attitude and Style* by Meg Mathews.

For when you feel you're being a shoddy parent and could do better: *The Book You Wish Your Parents Had Read* by Phillipa Perry.

If you want to learn more about past trauma: *The Body Keeps the Score: Mind, Brain and Body in the Transformation of Trauma* by Bessel van der Kolk.

For grief: *A Manual for Heartache* by Cathy Rentzenbrink; *Grief is the Thing with Feathers* by Max Porter; *A Year of Magical Thinking* by Joan Didion.

For when your knees are knocking together: *Feel the Fear and Do It Anyway* by Susan Jeffers.

If you want inspiration to run more often: *Running Like a Girl* by Alexandra Heminsley.

Podcasts

For gloomy days when you need a lift: 'The Adam Buxton podcast' with Adam Buxton.

For meditation and mindfulness advice: 'Tara Brach's podcast' with Tara Brach.

For grief: 'Griefcast' with Cariad Lloyd.

For culture and stuff that you're too tired to keep abreast with: 'The High Low' with Dolly Alderton and Pandora Sykes; 'Still Processing' with Wesley Morris and Jenna Wortham.

For sex and relationships: 'The Hotbed' with Lisa Williams, Anniki Sommerville and Cherry Healey.

For beginning to educate yourself about Black history in America: '1619' with Nikole Hannah-Jones (alongside other guest hosts).

For work inspiration: 'Work like a Woman' with Mary Portas.

For how to become an entrepreneur: 'In Good Company' with Otegha Uwagba.

For when you feel like a flop: 'How to Fail' with Elizabeth Day.

For when you need a laugh about the patriarchy: 'The Guilty Feminist' with Deborah Frances-White.

If you're ready to get sober or are sober-curious: 'Love Sober' with Kate & Mandy.

For when you're anxious: 'Unfuck Your Brain' with Kara Loewentheil; 'The Rich Roll Podcast' with Rich Roll.

For when you need some inspiration: 'Super Soul Conversations' with Oprah Winfrey. 'Unlocking Us' with Brené Brown.

If you need to learn more about institutionalised racism: 'About Race' with Reni Eddo- Lodge.

And a bit of a plug here... **For when you're ageing and don't know what to do about it:** 'How to Be a Boss at Ageing' with Anniki Sommerville.

Websites

For exercise: https://www.jemmashealthhub.com

For outdoor swimming: https://www.outdoorswimmingsociety.com/uk-wild-swimming-groups

For up-to-date menopause advice: Dr Louise Newson at https://www.menopausedoctor.co.uk

For advice on the psychological side of menopause: Dr Becky Quicke at https://www.beckyquicke.com

For advice and support on infertility: https://fertilitynetworkuk.org *and* https://www.fertilityfriends.co.uk

To find a counsellor: https://www.bacp.co.uk

For grief counselling: https://www.cruse.org.uk

For breathing exercises: https://www.youtube.com/watch?v=Oy4wvF9Z24A

For yoga: https://www.youtube.com/user/yogawithadriene

Instagram accounts

For advice on pregnancy after infertility and more: @tryingyears

For help and advice with menopause:
@megmathewsofficial_
@menopause_doctor

@thekarenarthur
@themenopausepsychologist
@theothersambaker

For beauty advice that isn't bull-crap: @salihughes

For tips on sober life and life coaching: @mandymannerscoach

For exercise: @jemmas_health_hub

For career, building your own business, life inspiration and more:
@emmagannonuk
@annie.auerbach
@mollyjanegunn

For motherhood, work and more:
@mother_pukka
@notsosmugnow
@helenwearsasize18
@candicebrathwaite
@mumologist

For design and fashion:
@knickers_models_own
@erica_davies
@stylemesunday

For comic relief: @bookofmum

For financial help and advice: @myfrugalyear

For down-to-earth humour/recommendations and more:
@cherryhealey

For advice on how to talk to children about race and more:
@drpragyaagarwal

To shape your education around race: @oteghauwagba
For inspiration around mysticism and more: @mysticalthinking

For tangible and pragmatic sex advice: @thesexdoctor *and* @thehotbedcollective

For inspirational art: @london_artist1

For writing and advice on surviving grief: @cariadlloyd

For mental health advice and tips: @hilda_burke_psychotherapist

And for inspiration, nostalgia, book and podcast reviews, menopause tips, and anything age-related, why not join the 'How to Be a Boss at Ageing' Facebook group?

ACKNOWLEDGEMENTS

I'd like to thank Paul, my partner, and my daughters Rae and Greta. They have all been super-patient when I've been hunched over my laptop, typing away. Also, thank you to my mum, step-dad John, step-mum Marylyn and sisters Camille, Sophie and Kate. And to all my friends who have encouraged me and helped me stay motivated. To all the people who agreed to be interviewed and helped with their advice and tips. And, finally, to the mums in the sandy park who offered up their thoughts, advice and challenges and helped shape the book.

And to all women who are struggling in their forties and looking for reasons to be optimistic, I see you, I salute you. You've got this.

Lightning Source UK Ltd.
Milton Keynes UK
UKHW010103240221
379241UK00002BA/174